Percutaneous Renal Surgery

David R Webb

Percutaneous Renal Surgery

A Practical Clinical Handbook

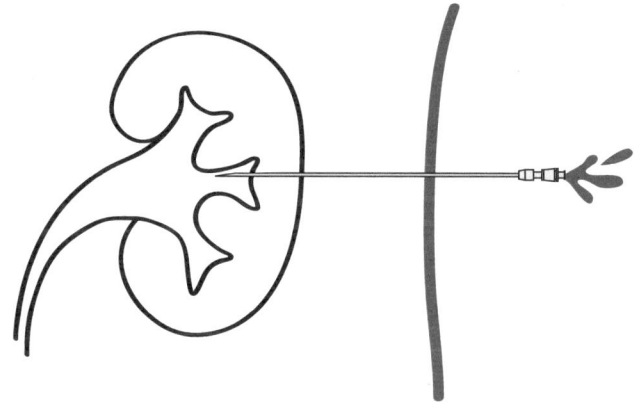

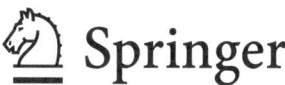

David R Webb
Surgery
University of Melbourne
Parkville
Victoria
Australia

ISBN 978-3-319-22827-3   ISBN 978-3-319-22828-0 (eBook)
DOI 10.1007/978-3-319-22828-0

Library of Congress Control Number: 2015957389

Springer Cham Heidelberg New York Dordrecht London
© Springer International Publishing Switzerland 2016
This work is subject to copyright. All rights are reserved by the Publisher, whether the whole or part of the material is concerned, specifically the rights of translation, reprinting, reuse of illustrations, recitation, broadcasting, reproduction on microfilms or in any other physical way, and transmission or information storage and retrieval, electronic adaptation, computer software, or by similar or dissimilar methodology now known or hereafter developed.
The use of general descriptive names, registered names, trademarks, service marks, etc. in this publication does not imply, even in the absence of a specific statement, that such names are exempt from the relevant protective laws and regulations and therefore free for general use.
The publisher, the authors and the editors are safe to assume that the advice and information in this book are believed to be true and accurate at the date of publication. Neither the publisher nor the authors or the editors give a warranty, express or implied, with respect to the material contained herein or for any errors or omissions that may have been made.

Printed on acid-free paper

Springer International Publishing AG Switzerland is part of Springer Science+Business Media (www.springer.com)

Preface

It is more than 30 years since the first elective endoscopic percutaneous removal of a calculus, initially via an operatively created nephrostomy and later via a radiologically established nephrostomy track (Alken et al. 1981).

Within 12 months this technique was embraced throughout Europe, America and Australia (Wickham and Kellett 1981).

I was fortunate to be the assistant at the first Australian percutaneous nephrolithotomy (PCNL) at the Royal Melbourne Hospital in 1982.

Extracorporeal shockwave lithotripsy (ESWL) was first performed in West Germany in 1980 by Professor Christian Chaussey (Chaussey et al. 1980).

Early ESWL required expensive technology and bulky equipment. As a result, ESWL was unavailable outside West Germany until John Wickham established the London Stone Centre in 1984 (Wickham et al. 1985).

In 1993 I had the privilege to work as senior urological registrar for the late Professor John Fitzpatrick, who introduced PCNL to Ireland, at the Meath Hospital, Dublin.

Under his supervision I studied the effects of PCNL on the canine kidney at Trinity College, Dublin, for my master of surgery thesis (Webb 1985).

Using these models, we demonstrated that a large nephrostomy could be created safely and established the anatomical basis for safe percutaneous access to the kidney (Webb and Fitzpatrick 1985).

These studies were confined to the kidney, its vasculature and the collecting system. They did not include the body wall.

Percutaneous radiological puncture of the kidney was routine for German trained urologists because they performed their own imaging.

However, most urologists outside Germany were not familiar with renal imaging, so a partnership was required between an interventional radiologist and urologist to create the nephrocutaneous access track.

Urologist–radiologist teams sprouted like mushrooms worldwide: Wickham and Kellett (UK), Fitzpatrick and Hurley (Ireland), Marberger and Hruby (Austria), Nunn and Hare (Melbourne), Segura and Castaneda (USA), etc. These partnerships developed the "two-stage percutaneous nephrolithotomy".

The first stage, the nephrostomy, was performed by the radiologist in the X-ray department on an awake patient.

The second, or endoscopic stage, was performed in the operating suite under general anaesthetic by the urologist, often many days after the nephrostomy.

This cumbersome, yet revolutionary, leap forward in removing renal calculi, was immediately successful for the removal of small renal stones.

It soon became apparent that these small stones were also the most suitable for contact-free ESWL. Experience quickly demonstrated that for the totally minimally invasive removal of all renal calculi, skills in both ESWL and PCNL were required (Webb et al. 1991).

Calculi most suitable for PCNL were hard, branched and infected stones associated with complex renal anatomy and compromised drainage.

Therefore, for these complex stones, the "two-stage" technique that utilised a single radiological track was inadequate to completely clear branched calculi.

This reality made it obvious that urologists practising PCNL for complex calculi had to be able to create their own separate nephrostomies at the time of surgery to achieve complete stone clearance.

The century-old skills of endoscopy were familiar to all urologists, but ultrasound and image intensifier (II) screening, and percutaneous renal puncture, were foreign concepts.

Urologists were not initially comfortable with a procedure they could not see!

In his keynote address to the Third World Congress of Percutaneous Surgery and ESWL (1985 New York), Professor Peter Alken summarised safe percutaneous access as "the shortest straight track entering the tip of a calyx". This "percutaneous epiphany" embodied our research and recommendations for safe intrarenal access. Alken's paradigm also included the track from the skin to the kidney.

In 30 years of practising and teaching percutaneous renal surgery (PCRS), it has been my experience that the major difficulty urologists experience with PCNL is that of percutaneous access.

There are no texts dedicated solely to renal access. Most descriptions are contained in large general endourological tomes. They tend to be confined to straightforward cases, rather than complex scenarios and options when an approach fails.

This manual aims to provide a simple "cookbook" for PCNL. It describes techniques for percutaneous renal access, attempting to demystify, explain and provide surgical plans to treat simple and complex calculi.

As a practical clinical handbook, this text is not an encyclopaedic reference book. Hence, instead of heavily referencing each chapter, I have provided a reading list at the end of the book. It combines 30 years of practice, teaching, research, international meetings and feedback from my colleagues and students and support from the University of Melbourne and especially Austin Health Melbourne. I was extremely fortunate to be in Europe during the embryonic years of PCNL and acknowledge the influences of John Wickham, John Fitzpatrick, Ron Miller,

Mike Kellett, Peter Alken and Michael Marberger and from the other side of the Atlantic, Joe Segura, Ralph Clayman, Arthur Smith, James Lingeman and countless others.

I could not have put my experiences on paper without the Austin Hospital supporting my sabbatical leave and the help of their theatre staff.

In this manual I generally describe my own technique, using a "single-stage dilator" (SSD), which has evolved over 30 years from our original and adapted concepts and experience and SSD access to the kidney was pioneered in Melbourne both clinically and in the laboratory.

The safety and development of this dilator was undertaken in 1991 in Melbourne as a prelude to the adaption of adult percutaneous renal surgery to infants and toddlers at the Royal Children's Hospital (Travis et al. 1991).

I use this dilator for every percutaneous renal operation but freely acknowledge that, as with all surgeons, each has their own favourite instrument and technique.

I do not claim the single-stage dilator to be superior to other methods of renal access. It is the instrument and technique that works best for me.

The concepts and methods described in this manual are equally transferable to the other commonly used systems including the serial Amplatz, balloon, telescoping metal dilators and the new single-stage dilators used with the miniature nephroscope system, commonly known as "mini perc".

This book does not attempt to be a textbook of endourology, but rather a series of simple algorithms for obtaining safe intrarenal access and stone clearance.

This manual is dedicated to my mentors, teachers and students, in particular Professor John Fitzpatrick, Mr John Wickham, Dr Michael Kellett and Professor Bill Hare and my Melbourne colleagues, Dr Trung Pham, Professor Damien Bolton, my fellow Austin Hospital urologists and theatre staff and, in particular, Professor Nathan Lawrentschuk who has never given up encouraging me to document my experience with PCRS.

This publication would not have been possible without the enormous advice and support of my co-author, Dr Olivia Herdiman; proof readers, Drs Frank Darcy and Rustom Mahecksha; and the magnificent illustrations by Jeffrey Gunadi BA. I owe them all my most profound gratitude.

Associate Professor David R Webb, MB, BS (Melb),
DRCOG (Eng), MS, MD (Melb), FRACS (Urol)
Associate Professor of Surgery
University of Melbourne
University Department of Surgery
Consultant Urological Surgeon
Department of Urology Austin Health Urologist
Royal Children's Hospital Urologist
Royal Australian Air Force (RAAFSR)
Parkville, VIC, Australia

References

Alken P, Hutschenreiter G, Gunther R, Marberger M (1981) Percutaneous stone manipulation. J Urol 125:463–466

Chaussey C, Brendel W, Schmidt E (1980) Extra corporeally induced destruction of kidney stones by shockwaves. Lancet 2:1265–1268

D'Arcy FT, Lawrentschuk N, Manecksha RP, Webb DR (2015) Renal track creation for percutaneous nephrolithotomy: the history and relevance of single stage dilation. Can J Urol. 22(5):7978–7983

Travis DG, Tan HL, Webb DR (1986) Single increment dilatation percutaneous renal surgery – an experimental study. Br J Urol 68:144–147

Webb DR (1985) A structural and functional analysis of nephrostomy and lithotripsy in the upper urinary tract (Master's thesis). University of Melbourne, Melbourne

Webb DR, Fitzpatrick JM (1985) Percutaneous nephro lithotripsy: a functional and morphological study. J Urol 134:587–591

Webb DR, Payne SR, Wickham JEA (1991) Extracorporeal shockwave lithotripsy and percutaneous renal surgery: comparisons, combinations, and conclusions. Br J Urol 58:1–5

Wickham JEA, Kellett MJ (1981) Percutaneous nephrolithotomy. Br J Urol 53:297–299

Wickham JEA, Webb DR, Payne SR, Kellett MJ, Watkinson G, Whitfield HN (1985) Extra corporeal shockwave lithotripsy: the first 50 patients treated in Britain. Br Med J 290:1188–1189

Suggested further reading

Patel U, Ghani K, and Anson K (2006) Endourology – A Practical Handbook. Taylor and Francis

Payne SR, Webb DR (1988) Percutaneous Renal Surgery. Churchill Livingstone

Smith AD, Preminger G, Badlani G, Kavoussi LR (2012) Smith's Textbook of Endourology. BC Decker Inc

Contents

1	**Applied Anatomy for Percutaneous Access**	1
	Anatomy	1
	Renal	1
	Good Track	10
	Bad Track	11
	The Body Wall	12
	Lumbodorsal Fascia	15
	Horseshoe Kidney	16
	Anatomy of the Horseshoe Kidney	16
2	**Personnel and Equipment**	19
	Medical Personnel	19
	Equipment Requirements	20
	Operation Table	20
	Patient Positioning	20
	Imaging	21
	C-ARM	21
	Access	22
	Hydrophilic or "Slippery" Guide Wires	22
	Artery Forceps	23
	Retrograde Catheter	23
	Urethral Catheter	23
	Patient Drape	26
	Bairhugger: Blankets and Drapes	26
	Antibiotics	26
	DVT: Prophylaxis	26
	Scalpel	27
	Guide Wires	27
	Guide Wires-Types	27
	Nephrostomy Track Dilators	28
	Characteristics of Various Dilators	28

Amplatz Sheath	32
Puncture Needle	35
Irrigation Fluid	36
Nephroscopes	36
Instruments for Intracorporal Stone Fragmentation	37
Pneumatic Ballistic Lithotrites (Lithoclast)	37
Sonotrode	38
Equipment for Percutaneous Endoscopic Pyloplasty (or Endopyelotomy)	39
Stone Grasping Instruments	40
Graspers	40
Nephrostomies	42
Cope Nephrostomy	44
Foley Balloon Catheters	44
Other Drain Tubes	45
Tubeless Nephrostomy	46
Chest Drains	46

3 Indications for PCNL 47
    Introduction 47
    Options for the Treatment of Renal Calculi 48
    Indications for PCNL 48
    Current Indications for PCNL 49
    Contraindications to PCNL 49
    Schematic Comparison of ESWL and PCNL 50
        ESWL 50
    Preoperative Investigations Prior to PCNL 51
        Summary: Preoperative Investigations for PCNL ... 52
    Consent 52
        Preoperative Theatre Preparation 52

4 Percutaneous Nephrostomy 55
    Percutaneous Nephrostomy (PCN) 55
        Surgical Nephrostomy (SN) 55
        Skinny Needle Surgical Nephrostomy (SNSN) 55
        Radiological Nephrostomy (RN) 56
    Surgical Nephrostomy 56
        Puncture Technique 56
    Parallax 58
        Step 1 58
    Technique of Percutaneous Renal Puncture 64
        Lithotomy Position 64
        Prone Position of the Patient 66
        Theatre Set-Up 68
    Radiological Nephrostomy 81
        Definition 81

5 Routine PCNL ... 83

- Track Dilatation ... 83
- Track Size ... 84
- Track Dilatation ... 84
  - Aim ... 84
  - Principles ... 84
  - Kinked Guide Wire ... 86
  - The Body Wall Component of the Nephrostomy Track ... 87
  - The Skin ... 87
  - Lumbodorsal Fascia ... 87
- Track Dilation ... 88
  - Guide Wire ... 88
  - Dilator ... 88
- Commencement of the Track and Kidney Dilation ... 89
- Nephroscopy and Stone Removal ... 90
  - Plan ... 90
  - Nephroscopes ... 91
  - Blood Clots ... 92
  - Clot Removal ... 93
- Universal Guide Wire ... 93
  - The Creation of a Universal Guide Wire ... 94
  - Advantages of a Universal Guide Wire ... 96
- Stone Fragmentation ... 97
  - Alternative Energy Sources for Stone Fragmentation ... 97
  - Optimal Lithotrites for Stone Fragmentations ... 97
  - Aims of Stone Fragmentation ... 97
  - The Sonotrode ... 98
  - Choice of Lithotrite ... 99
- Stone Extraction for PCNL ... 100
- Stone Clearance ... 103
- Assessment of Stone Clearance at PCNL ... 104
- Nephrostomy Post PCNL ... 104
- Nephrostomy Types ... 104
  - "Cope" Loop Nephrostomy ... 105
  - Foley Catheter ... 105
  - Tube Nephrostomy (Splinted) ... 105
  - Tubeless Nephrostomy ... 106
- Technique of "Cope" Nephrostomy Insertion Following PCNL ... 106
- Alternative Method of Insertion of the "Cope"
- Loop Nephrostomy ... 107
- Lost Nephrostomy ... 108
- Suturing the "Cope" Nephrostomy Tube to the Skin ... 108
  - Technique of Cope Nephrostomy Suture ... 109
- Post-operative Care of the Nephrostomy ... 109
  - Nephrostogram ... 110

6	**Complex PCNL and Antegrade Endopyelotomy**	111
	Complex Calculi	111
	Complex Anatomy	112
	Introduction	115
	Advanced Skills Required for Difficult PCNL	115
	Scenario One: Large Infection-related Staghorn Calculus	115
	Aim	115
	Potential Problems	116
	Preoperative Tests, Treatment and Precautions	116
	CT-IVP	116
	Pyonephrosis	117
	Difficulties Encountered with Punctures for Complete Staghorn Calculi	118
	Technique of Creating an Endoscopic Nephrotomy	125
	Supplementary Target Punctures during Staghorn Calculus Removal	129
	Scenario Two: Complex Recurrent Infection Calculi Associated with a Chronically Infected Urinary Diversion or Associated Neurogenic Bladder	135
	Indications for Stone Removal	135
	Theatre: Additional Equipment	136
	Scenario Three: Calculi Within Calyceal Diverticulae	137
	Anticipated Difficulties	137
	Aims of the Puncture for Treatment of Stones in a Calyceal Diverticulum	138
	Preparation Prior to Surgery for Calculi in Calyceal Diverticulae	138
	"Y" Puncture Technique	141
	Stone Removal from a Calyceal Diverticulum	144
	Drainage	144
	Scenario Four: The Management of Calculi in a Narrow or Poorly Draining Calyx, or a Stone Forming a Complete Cast of a Calyx	146
	Scenario Five	146
	Previous Renal Surgery	146
	Renal Scarring	147
	Summary of the Management of Patient Undergoing PCNL in the Presence of Significant Renal and Perirenal Scarring	147
	Scenario Six	147
	Obese Patients	147
	Preoperative Planning	148
	Scenario Seven	150
	Horseshoe Kidney	150
	Preoperative Planning	150

Scenario Eight... 151
  Large-Impacted Pelviureteric Junction and/or Upper
  Ureteric Calculus 151
  Large Upper Ureteric Calculus 152
  Plan for Antegrade PCNL to Remove a Large Upper
  Ureteric Calculus 152
  Preoperative Planning 152
  The "Three-Wire" Antegrade Ureteroscopy Technique......... 157
  Amplatz Trauma.. 159
Scenario Nine 161
  Percutaneous Puncture of a Large Hydronephrosis 161
Scenario Ten: Percutaneous Endopyelotomy (Pyeloplasty).... 161
  Indications 161
  Surgical Points of Technique and Difficulties
  with Percutaneous Endopylotomy 162
  Operative Plan 162
  Percutaneous Endopyelotomy: Operative Technique.......... 166
  Precautions... 167

7 Complications of PCNL 169
Introduction... 169
Anatomical Factors Related to PCNL Complications 169
  The Kidney.. 169
  Blood Supply 170
  Collecting System 170
  Access to the Kidney Is Blind 170
  Intrarenal Anatomy 171
  Summary 171
Complications Related to the Nephrostomy Puncture 172
  Guide Wire Kinking During Dilation...................... 172
Damage to Neighbouring Organs 172
  Bowel... 172
  Needle Puncture of the Bowel 173
  Dilator Trauma to the Bowel 173
  Renal Vein or IVC Puncture.............................. 175
Complications During Track Dilation........................ 175
  Lost Track During Dilation 175
  If You Are Unable to Successfully Puncture a Selected Calyx 176
Amplatz Trauma... 176
  Sites of Amplatz Sheath Trauma 177
  Lost Amplatz Sheath 178
Forceps Trauma... 178
  Triradiate Forceps...................................... 178

Renal Pelvis Perforation 179
    Management of a Large Pelvic or Infundibular Tear 180
    Management of Complete PUJ Avulsion 180
Infundibular Tears 180
    Sonotrode Trauma 180
    "Lost" Calculi 181
    Lost Nephrostomy Track 182
Urinary Tract Infection and Septicaemia 182
    Management 182
Pneumothorax 183
Bleeding 183
Residual Calculi 184
DVT 185

Appendix I: Critical Pathways, Theatre Equipment Lists and Setups ... 187
  Equipment and Set-Up for PCNL (Nurses Set Up Notes
  for A/Prof D. Webb Theatre) 187
    Cystoscopy Trolley 187
    General Trolley (Top) 188
    Drains and Dressings 188
    For Endoscopic Pyeloplasty/Endopyelotomy 189
    Positioning for Patients with Skeletal Deformities
    and Spinal Cord Injury 189
  Nurse Information for PCNL 189
    Information Sheet 189
  Post-operative Patient Instructions 191
    Going Home After Your PCNL 191
    Comfort and Pain 191
    Dressing 191
    Medications 192
    Activity 192
    Hygiene 192
    Nutrition 192
    Returning to Work and Driving 192
    Consent Form 193
    Risks 193
    Normal Results 194

Appendix II: PCNL Workshop 195
  Workstations 195
  Participants 196
  Materials Required for This Workshop 196
    Equipment for Workshop 5 197

Stations
- Station 1: The Surgical Anatomy of the Kidney and Collecting System Related to Percutaneous Renal Surgery (PCRS) 197
- Station 2: The Surgical Anatomy of the Kidney and Collecting System Relating to the Establishment of a PCRS Track 201
- Station 3: Techniques for Difficult Renal Punctures and Renal Access 216
- Station 4: Trauma to the Kidney, Renal Vessels and Collecting System during PCNL 223
- Station 5: Percutaneous Nephrolithotomy – Endoscopic Stone Fragmentation and Equipment 232

Glossary and Definitions 249

Index 255

About the Author

Associate Professor David Webb graduated from the University of Melbourne, Australia and completed his urological training (FRACS-Urology) at the Royal Melbourne Hospital. He gained postgraduate experience with Mr J E A Wickham at the Institute of Urology, London, and Professor John Fitzpatrick at the Meath Hospital, Dublin.

His master of surgery thesis (Trinity College Dublin and the University of Melbourne) evaluated the anatomical and pathophysiological effects of percutaneous nephrostomy and nephrolithotripsy on the kidney.

His doctor of medicine thesis (University of Melbourne) described the development of a number of instruments for percutaneous renal surgery, particularly, the Webb "single-stage dilator". His papers include the evolution of the combination of extracorporeal shockwave lithotripsy and percutaneous renal surgery and the development of percutaneous renal surgery and the SSD for the management of paediatric and adult calculi.

Associate Professor Webb has conducted endourological workshops in the United Kingdom, Vietnam, Indonesia, Myanmar, the Royal Australasian College of Surgeons and at numerous Scientific Meetings of the Urological Society of Australia and New Zealand, and the Societe Internationale d'Urologiu (SIU).

He is currently associate professor of surgery at the University of Melbourne and consultant urologist to Austin Health, Melbourne; the Royal Children's Hospital, Melbourne; and the Royal Australian Air Force.

Chapter 1
Applied Anatomy for Percutaneous Access

It is essential to have a basic knowledge of renal surgical anatomy, in particular the capsule, renal parenchyma, collecting system and vasculature.

The track for PCRS access is comprised of two components, the extrarenal (or body wall) and renal.

Anatomy

Renal

The renal parenchyma is encased by a thin firm, fibrous capsule.

The capsule is felt by a slight resistance and then a "give" when the kidney is punctured by the access needle.

Once the needle is within the parenchyma, it will move externally with respiration.

The collecting system begins as calyces, which coalesce to form the infundibulum, renal pelvis, pelviureteric junction and ureter (Fig. 1.1).

The upper and lower pole calyces are usually compound; the mid zone calyces are simple. The calyces are directed anteriorly and posteriorly. The posterior calyces usually point about 30° backwards, so a puncture into a posterior calyx leads directly to the infundibulum and renal pelvis. The anterior calyces are directed more forward, so when punctured from behind, the entry is at an acute angle, which may be difficult to negotiate with dilators or rigid nephroscopes.

The only portion of the collecting system that is physically attached to the renal parenchyma is the outermost tip of the calyx at the fornix (Fig. 1.1). The infundibula and pelvis are unsupported and mobile.

It is logical and confirmed experimentally that the tip of the calyx is the safest and most appropriate entry site for percutaneous puncture and renal dilatation.

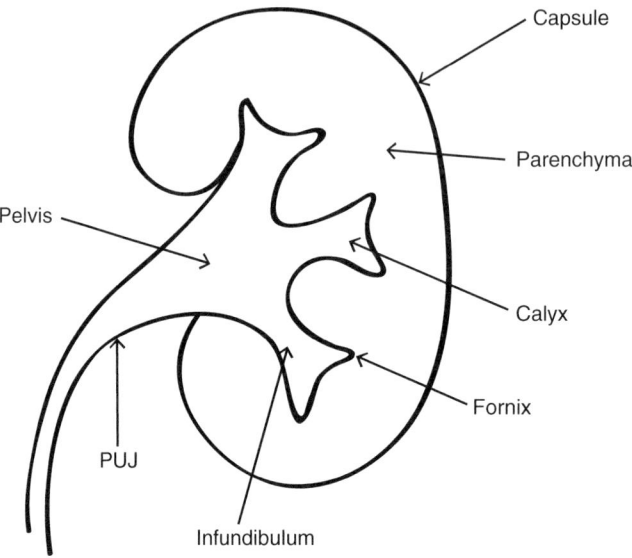

Fig. 1.1 Basic renal anatomy for PCNL

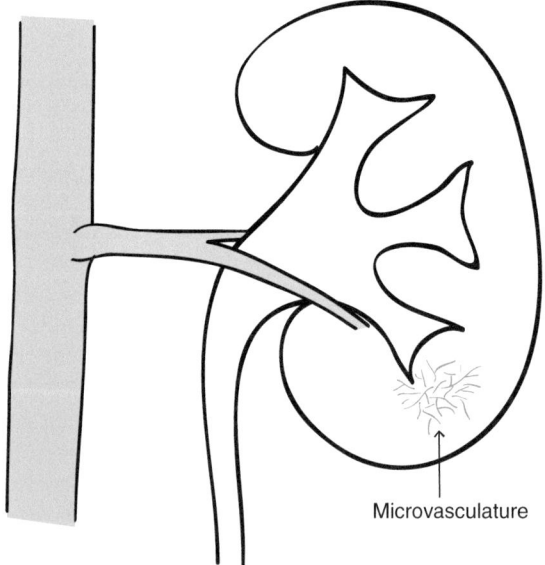

Fig. 1.2 The peripheral microvasculature of the kidney

Not only is this where the only portion of the collecting system is attached to the kidney, it is also the thinnest region of renal parenchyma where there are no large renal segmental vessels, only microvasculature (Fig. 1.1).

Anatomy

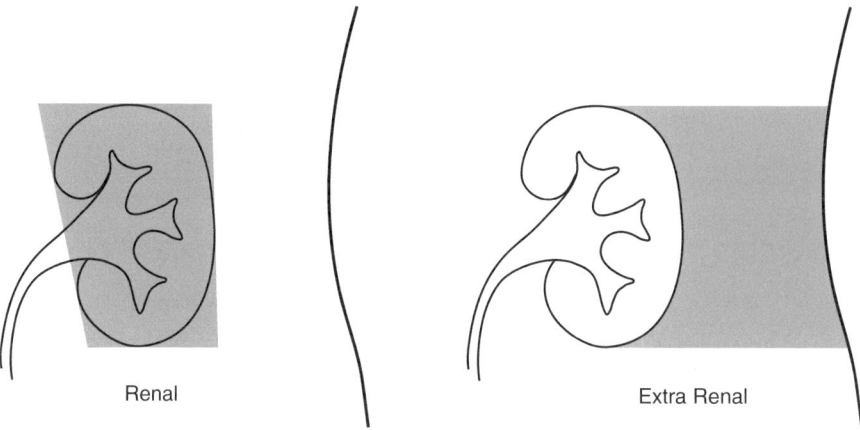

Fig. 1.3 The renal and extrarenal components of the PCNL track

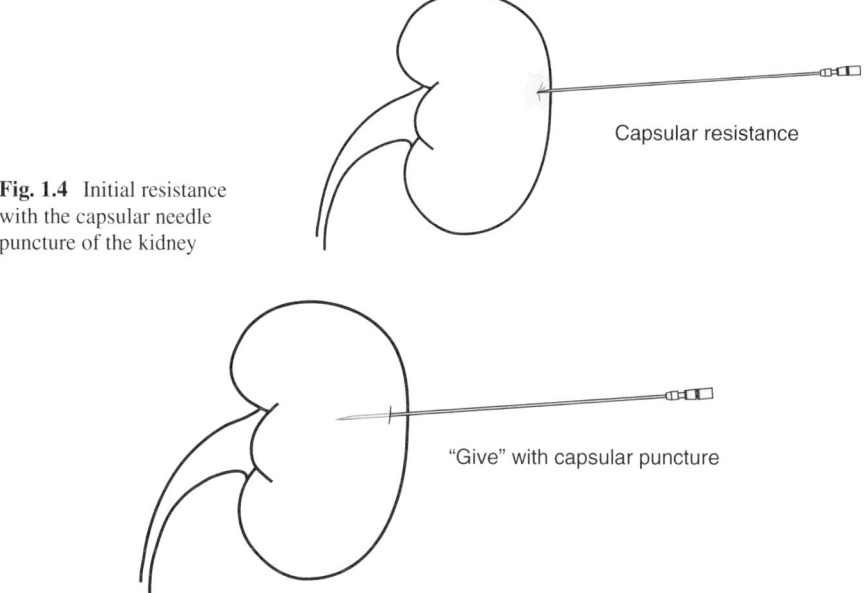

Fig. 1.4 Initial resistance with the capsular needle puncture of the kidney

Fig. 1.5 Perforation of the renal capsule by the needle puncture results in a sharp small advance, felt as the "give" sign

The renal segmental vessels are end arteries. As a result, damage to a segmental vessel can result in haemorrhage, arteriovenous fistula, pseudo-aneurysm, or segmental infarction.

There is no arterial cross circulation from one segment to another.

In contrast, the renal veins do communicate across segments, so venous injuries are less damaging.

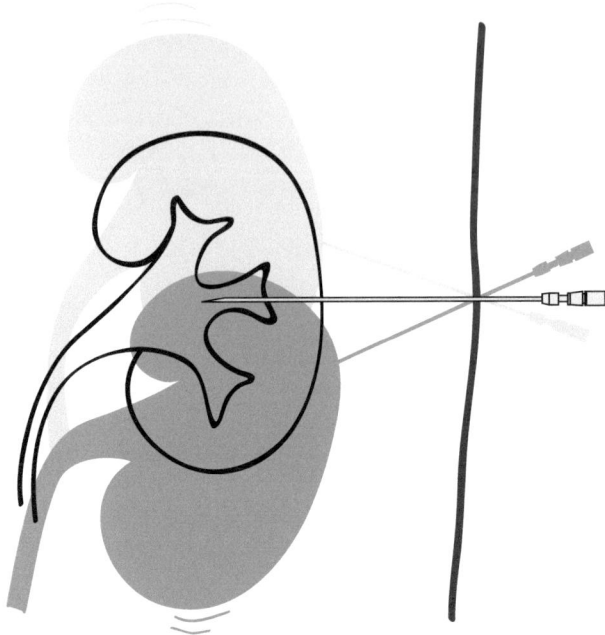

Fig. 1.6 External movement of the hub of the puncture needle with respiration once the needle tip has entered the kidney

However, as the peripheral renal parenchyma is only comprised of microvasculature and no major vessels, puncture and dilatation of this region does not cause significant vascular or renal damage.

Most percutaneous endoscopic instruments are rigid. It is logical that if they enter through the thinnest region of the kidney, intrarenal manipulation of the endoscope will occur across the narrowest fulcrum, causing the least amount of renal disruption.

By entering the kidney through the tip of a calyx, as an instrument advances centrally, it is separated from the segmental vessels by the collecting system and so cannot cause vascular damage.

The surgeon aims to introduce instruments within and parallel to the axis of the calyx so that they do not traumatise the collecting system or the adjacent segmental vessels.

The collecting system is muscular and dynamic.

The calyces, infundibula and renal pelvis contract.

When puncturing the kidney, "irritation" of the collecting system by the needle at the tip of the calyx can induce a "spastic contraction" of the calyx. This can often be appreciated when screening as "the half moon sign", in which a calyceal contraction or spasm will alter the distribution of contrast within the calyx, producing a crescent or "half moon" appearance.

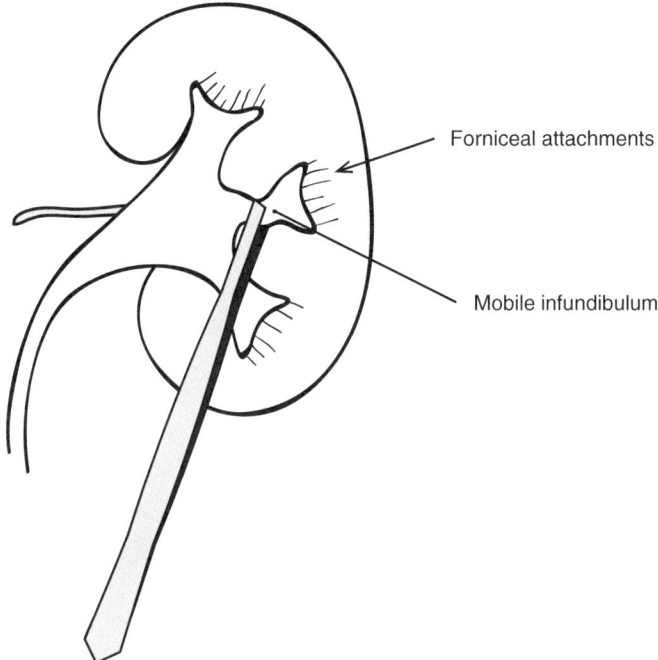

Fig. 1.7 The collecting system is only attached to the kidney at the fornices, elsewhere it is mobile. This is easily demonstrated on a bivalved cadaver kidney by grasping the infundibulum with dissecting forceps, as illustrated above

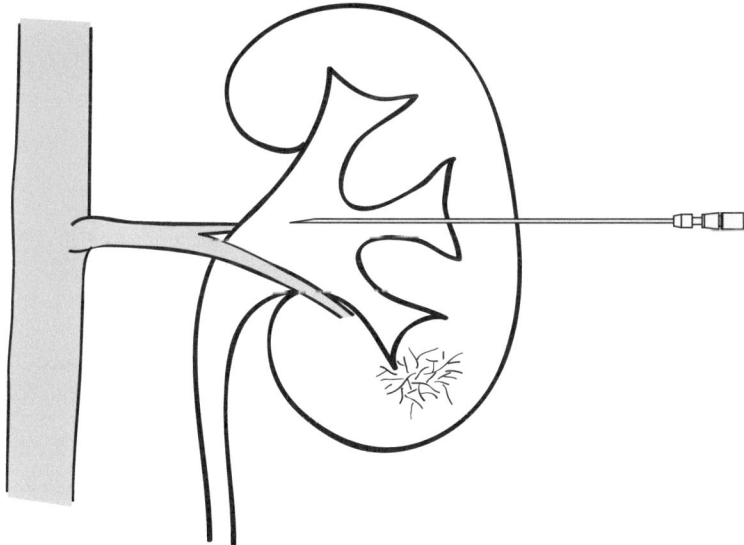

Fig. 1.8 Needle puncture entering the tip of a calyx

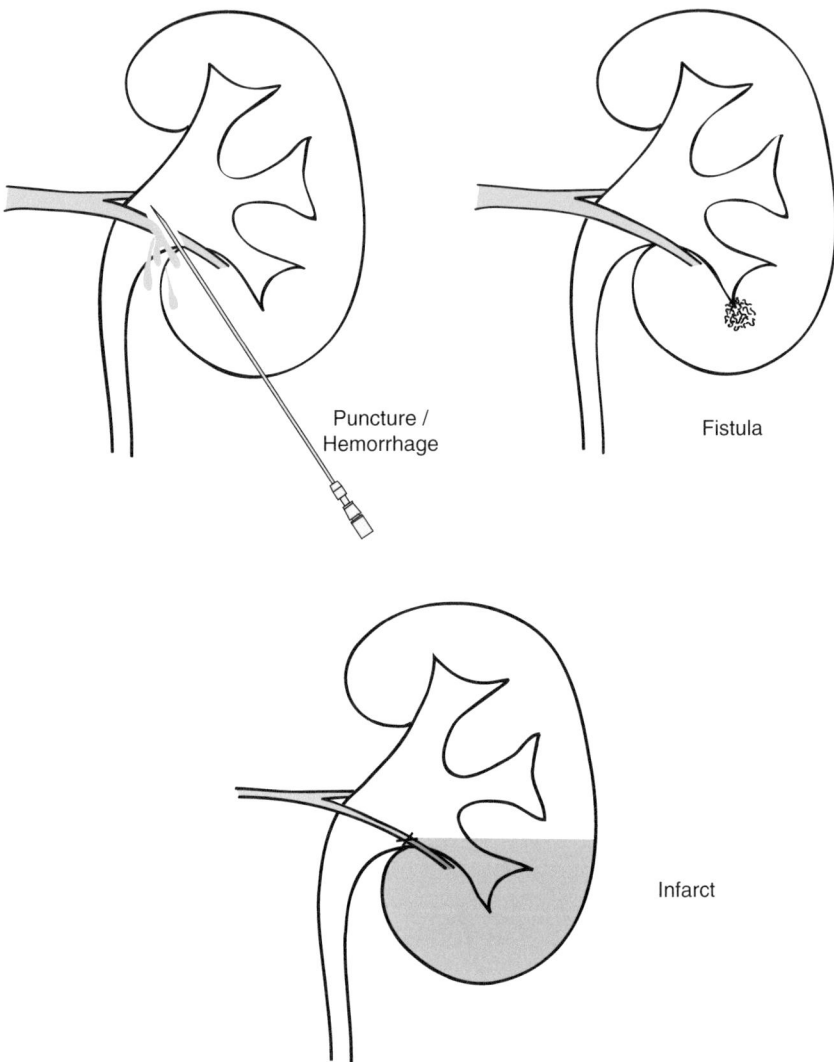

Fig. 1.9 Damage to a segmental renal artery causing haemorrhage, a fistula, or segmental infarction

When this spasm occurs, the needle tip is usually at the edge of the calyx, but not necessarily in the lumen. At this point, a very short advancement of the needle usually gains entry to the calyx and the lumen of the collecting system.

The kidney is a pedicled organ, surrounded by fat within Gerota's fascia. As a result, the kidney is very mobile, although limited to a degree as the major renal vessels are relatively short. It not only moves with the respiration but can also be displaced or rotated anteriorly during the puncture and dilation phase. This anterior displacement is exacerbated by the fact that the lower pole is already tilted forward, relative to the upper pole, as the kidney lies on the psoas and quadratus muscles.

Anatomy

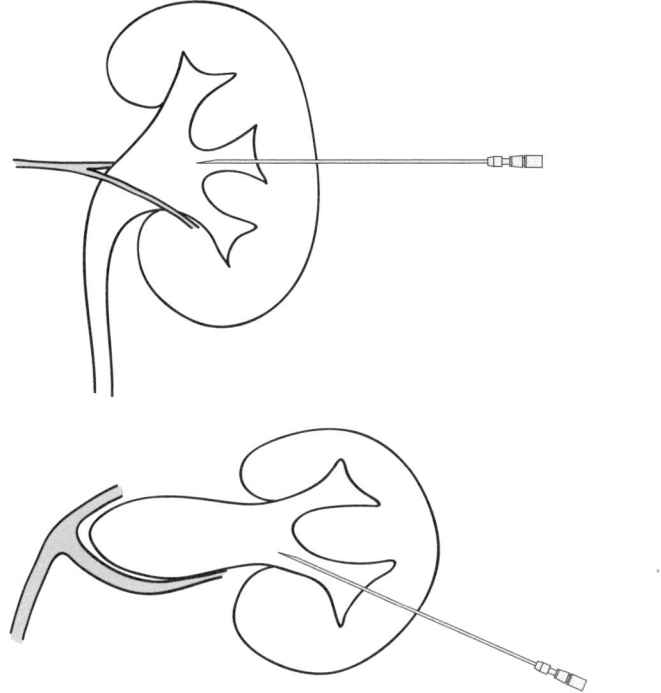

Fig. 1.10 Vertical (*top*) and transverse (*bottom*) sections through the site of a renal puncture

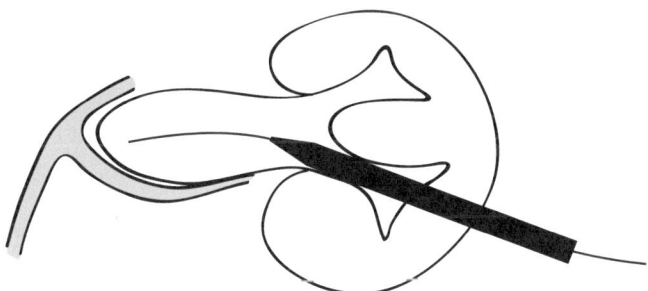

Fig. 1.11 Renal dilator entering the tip of a calyx over a guide wire

Once a track is established, the kidney will move with the instruments.

The surgeon needs to be aware of this mobility when accessing the collecting system. The urologist should always attempt to pass the guide wire through the calyx and down the ureter. This helps to stabilise and straighten the dilatation track.

Renal mobility and track instability are most marked at the upper and lower poles. This fact needs to be borne in mind with polar punctures, particularly those into calyceal diverticulae.

The renal capsule is easily penetrated by needles and dilators.

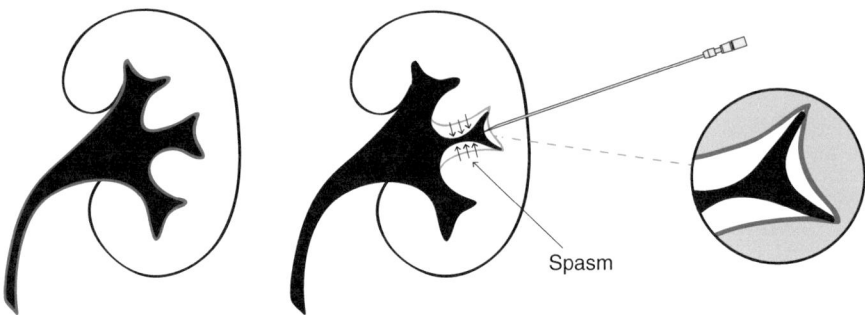

Fig. 1.12 Calyceal spasm and the "half moon sign"

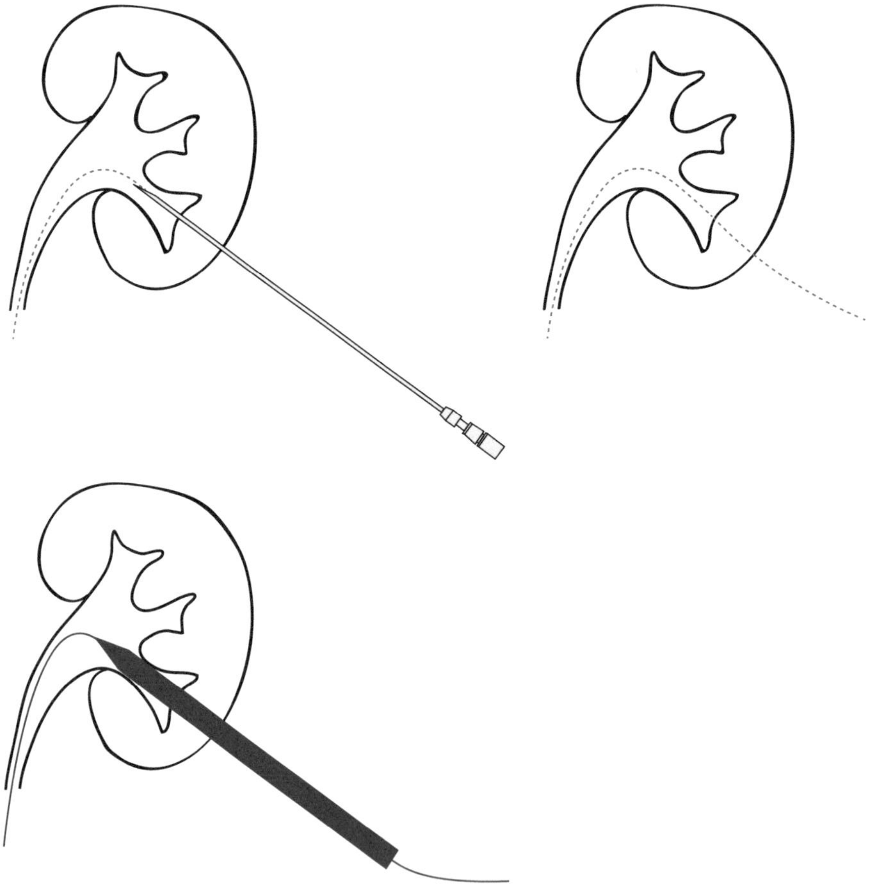

Fig. 1.13 Uncomplicated needle puncture followed by insertion of a guide wire and renal dilator, which passes atraumatically through the calyceal lumen

Anatomy

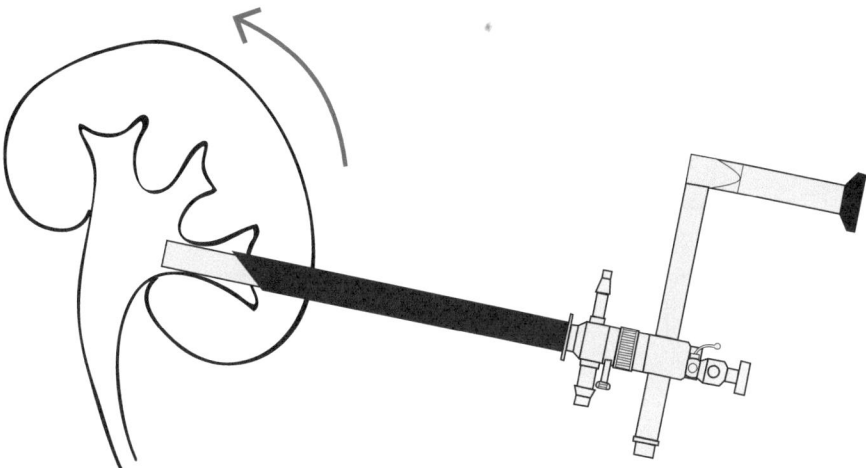

Fig. 1.14 The mobile kidney will move freely with nephroscope and sheath movements

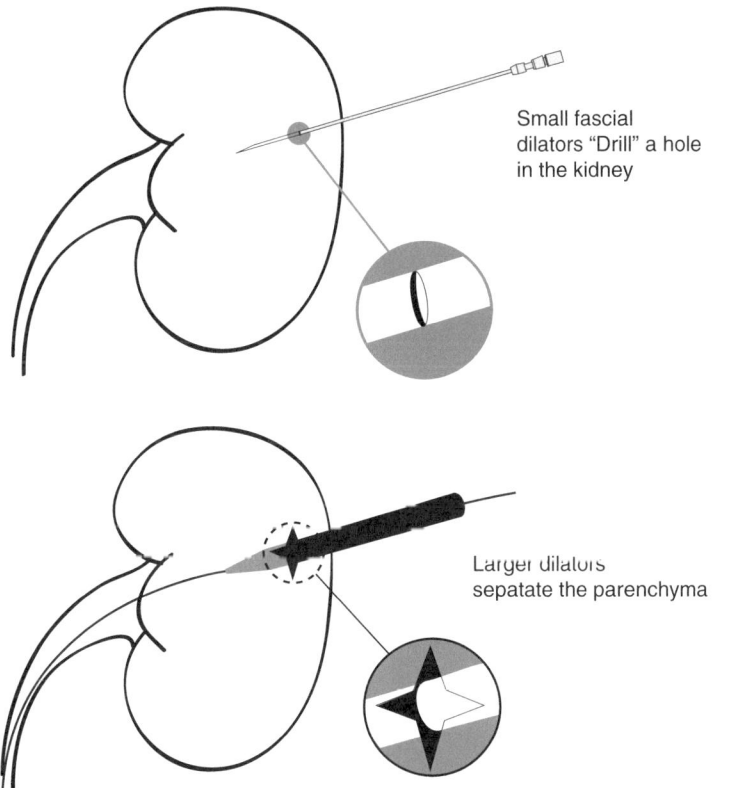

Fig. 1.15 The fascial dilators initially "drill" the parenchyma, the larger dilators separate the parenchyma, creating a nephrotomy

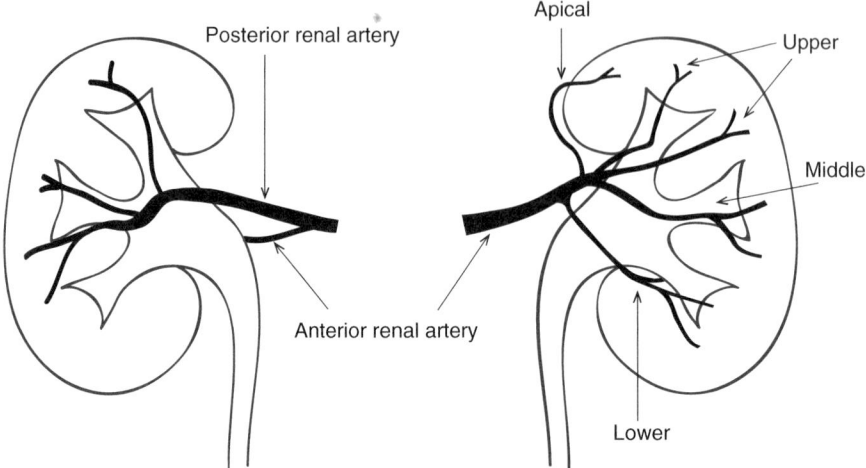

Fig. 1.16 The usual segmental renal blood supply

The parenchyma is solid but not particularly rigid. Small dilators "drill" a hole through the parenchyma until they reach about 12–14 Fr. Subsequent dilators separate the parenchymal track along and parallel to the lines of the pyramids.

Separation does not cause parenchymal damage, as it does not cut the kidney and is only in the region of microvasculature, not the segmental vessels.

In essence, it is the same process used in creating an open nephrotomy.

Renal arterial vasculature commonly varies. Usually, there is one renal artery arising from the aorta, with anterior and posterior divisions, four being anterior and one posterior.

An aberrant lower pole vessel occurs approximately 1 in 7. This may be implicated in reconstruction of the pelviureteric junction by an Anderson–Hynes pyeloplasty and must be borne in mind if contemplating an endoscopic pyeloplasty.

It is important to access the operative details of the previous pyeloplasty to confirm whether the renal artery is behind or in front of the repair, to avoid division of an anterior vessel during endopyelotomy.

Good Track

In summary, "the shortest straight track" that only traverses the microvasculature will result in minimal parenchymal disruption provided it enters through the tip of the calyx into and parallel to the collecting system.

Anatomy

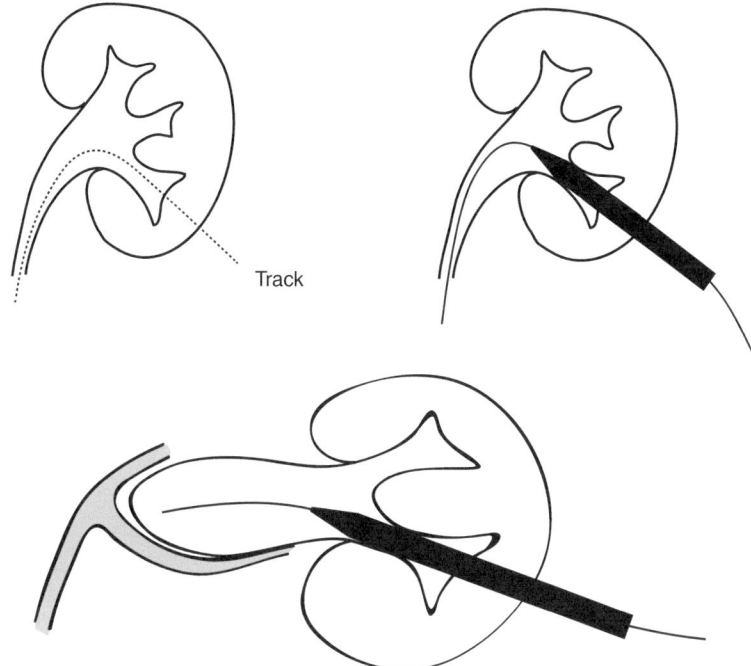

Fig. 1.17 The ideal puncture for renal dilation

Bad Track

Conversely, a track that does not follow these anatomical principles is prone to complications.

The longer a track is through the real parenchyma, the more the kidney will split with movement of the operative sheath and endoscope and so the less mobility the nephroscope will have within the kidney. This in turn compromises access to upper and lower poles and neighbouring calyces.

A longer track enters the kidney medially and so traverses the renal sinus, thereby directly endangering the major segmental vessels. This trauma can cause haemorrhage, infarction, AV fistula formation, pseudo-aneurysm, and may require emergency transfusion and radiological segmental artery embolisation.

Unsupported, the collecting system is more prone to tearing during dilatation and instrumentation. As a result, irrigant fluid will extravasate; the kidney will become displaced; the collecting system will collapse, resulting in poor vision with bleeding and extravasation of stone fragments outside the kidney.

In general, split renal parenchyma will close, tamponade and heal. If a medial puncture is noticed early, and the dilator removed, it is usually safe to continue and puncture another calyx.

However, if a large renal split or collecting system tear has occurred, the procedure should be abandoned and a nephrostomy and/or double J stent inserted.

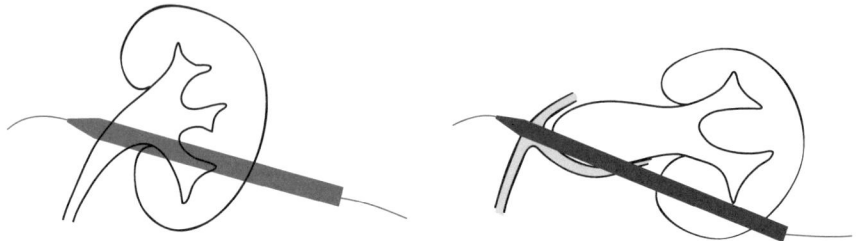

Fig. 1.18 Poor renal puncture

Unless there is significant vascular damage, the kidney will heal and a later elective PCNL can be planned.

The Body Wall

For most punctures, the layers traversed through the body wall are skin, subcutaneous fat, body wall muscle, lumbodorsal fascia, Gerota's fascia, perirenal fat, and occasionally the diaphragm, pleura, and intercostal spaces.

In the case of a horseshoe kidney, the puncture may transverse the vertical back muscles. Posteriorly, a horseshoe kidney usually has no adjacent organs, but occasionally, bowel may be present and must be excluded on preoperative imaging.

Anteriorly, the normal kidney is related to the liver, colon and duodenum on the right and the spleen, descending colon, duodenum on the left. Both the ascending and descending colon can lie posterior to the right and left kidney, most commonly the left lower pole, in about 15 % of patients. While very uncommon, an enlarged liver or spleen can extend lateral to the kidney.

The majority of punctures for PCNL enter the lower pole of the kidney, are infracostal, and enter the skin in the general region of the renal lumbar triangle.

However, for an upper pole puncture and high kidneys, it may be necessary for the puncture to be above the twelfth or even the eleventh rib.

The pleura lies below the medial aspect of the twelfth rib, and the majority of the inferior aspect of the eleventh rib.

It is essential for surgeons to be aware of this fact, and to check a CT of the abdomen and lower chest prior to any renal puncture.

The skin is a tough layer, is mobile, and is the only part of the operation that the patient sees.

Patients prefer the smallest scar.

The initial puncture should be made through a small 2–3 mm stab, which allows the needle and its sheath to pass through the skin without damage. The skin puncture site should not be enlarged until renal access is confirmed.

The smallest incision necessary should be made parallel to Langer's lines to reduce scar formation. A vertical skin incision will result in a very thick and ugly scar.

The Body Wall

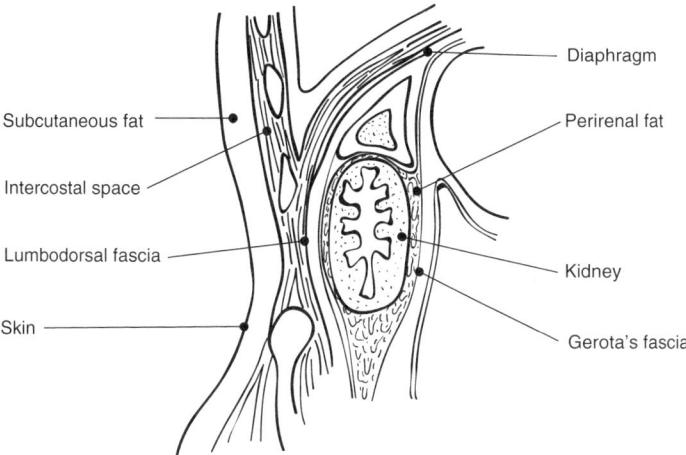

Fig. 1.19 Body wall anatomical relationships for PCNL

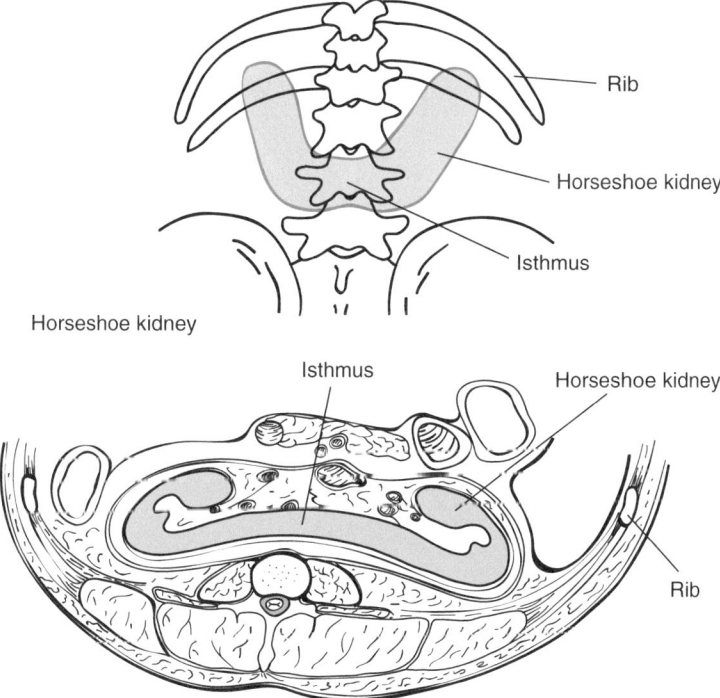

Fig. 1.20 Vertical and transverse sections showing the most common relationships of a horseshoe kidney

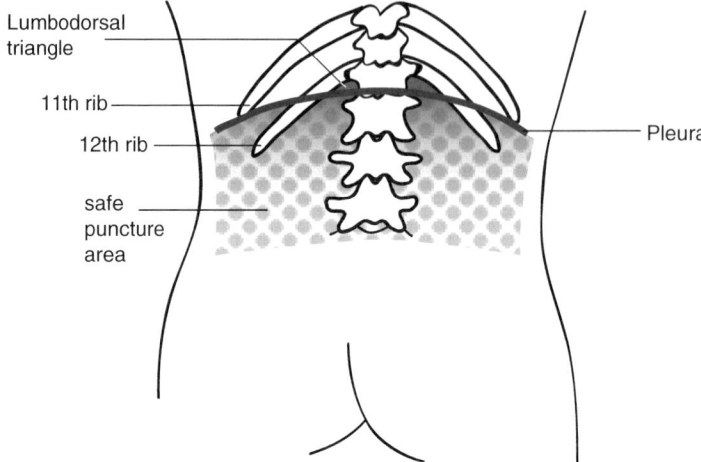

Fig. 1.21 The safe areas for puncture to avoid transgressing the pleura, the lumbar triangle lying above the twelfth rib

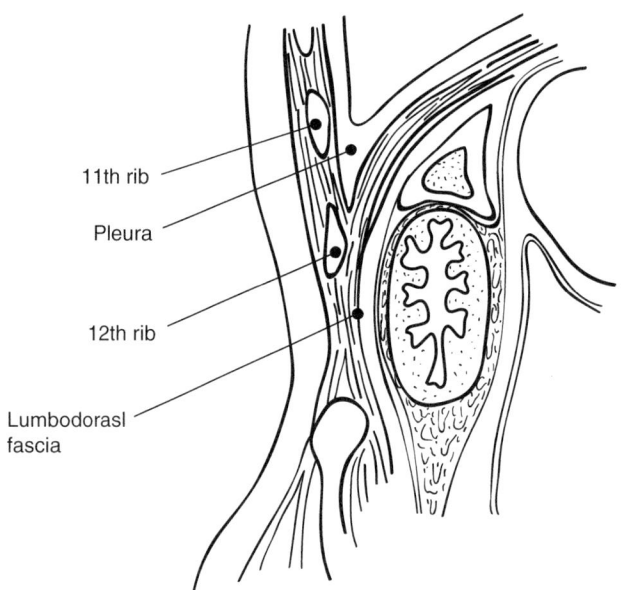

Fig. 1.22 The lateral reflections of the pleura related to the mid 12th rib and upper pole of the kidney

Ribs present a number of potential problems.

Firstly, although they may not appear to be in the line of the puncture on imaging, they still may obstruct the path of the needle.

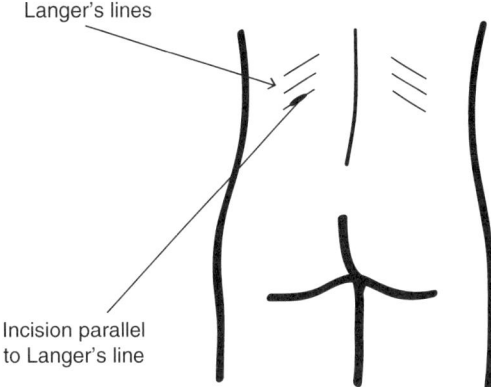

Fig. 1.23 The direction of Langer's line in the lumbar region

In that case, the puncture entry site needs to be moved.

The intercostal vessels and nerves travel directly below the rib and are vulnerable, so punctures should be made at the upper border of a rib if possible to avoid the neurovascular bundle. Intercostal spaces can be narrow, making insertion of the dilator difficult through a narrow and rigid space, especially medially.

Assuming that any puncture above a rib can potentially involve pleura, supracostal tracks should never be forcibly expanded with forceps or sharp instruments.

Even if it is not apparent to the surgeon that a supracostal puncture has traversed pleura, all patients must have a chest x-ray following PCRS if the puncture is above any rib.

Even so, only 3 % of supra 12 punctures result in a pneumothorax. As the lung is above the 11th rib, lung parenchymal injury is rare unless the puncture is above the 10th rib or higher.

Lumbodorsal Fascia

This is the densest plane in the flank through which the track passes.

It is the hardest layer to dilate, is rigid and tends to split, so that it may clamp down on instruments with a "scissoring effect".

Many stones that were attempted to be extracted outside the Amplatz sheath have become dislodged by this "scissoring" phenomenon and remain in the backs of patients.

As a result of this difficulty and rigidity, I open the lumbodorsal fascia with the tips of artery forceps under II guidance, prior to inserting the renal dilator, to decrease friction on the dilator and increase the sensitivity and feel during dilatation of the kidney.

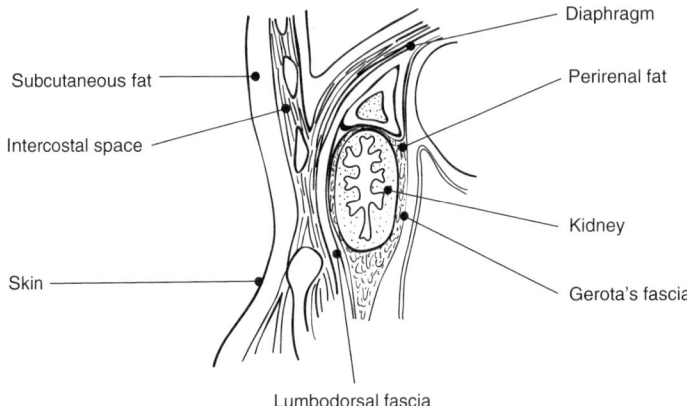

Fig. 1.24 The relationship of the lumbodorsal fascia to the back muscles and the kidney

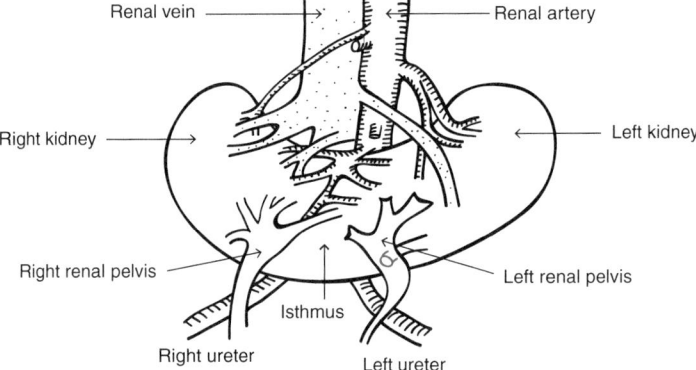

Fig. 1.25 Renal vascular and collecting system anatomy in a horseshoe kidney

Horseshoe Kidney

A horseshoe kidney is one that has been arrested in its ascent from the bony pelvis; the moieties are not fully rotated and are attached across the midline by a fibrous isthmus.

Anatomy of the Horseshoe Kidney

1. Vasculature
    Although different to the distribution in orthotopic renal anatomy, the vasculature of a horseshoe kidney rarely creates a surgical problem.
    The vessels come from behind and below the kidney, and unless one makes a puncture so medial that it would traverse the inferior vena cava or aorta, no

Horseshoe Kidney

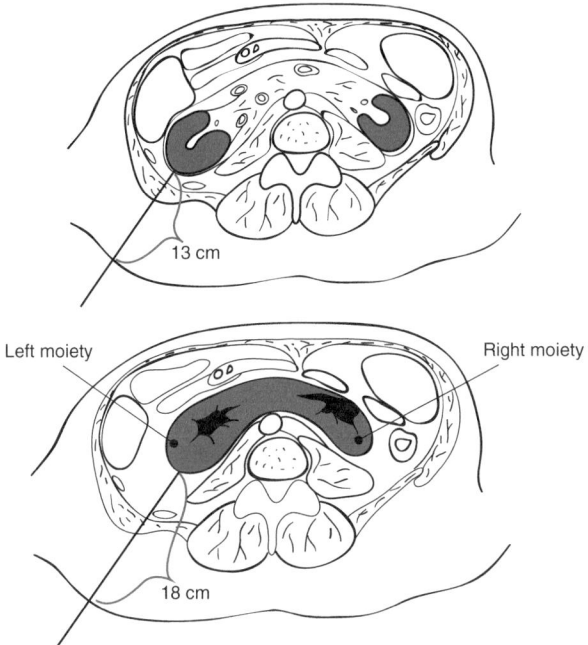

Fig. 1.26 Comparison of the body wall distance to an orthotopic (*top*) and horseshoe kidney (*bottom*)

significant vessels are encountered with percutaneous puncture of a horseshoe kidney.

2. Collecting system

   As the kidney has not fully rotated, the upper and outer calyces are malrotated and the medial calyces are often distorted. The medial calyces are particularly difficult to access from the renal pelvis with a rigid endoscope due to a combination of angulation and distance. Hence, when treating a horseshoe kidney one should include a flexible cystoscope and laser in the set-up. They are unfortunately the calyces often containing calculi as they are lower most

3. Pelvis and pelviureteric junction

   These are anterior and run up and over the isthmus, which may result in compromised drainage. The closest calyx in a horseshoe kidney to the skin is the most lateral and upper. It is also the furthest away from the renal pelvis and usually deep, 15–20 cm from the skin.

4. Paraspinal muscles – these are medial and may need to be traversed by the puncture, which can result in a rigid and a track that is difficult to dilate.

All patients with horseshoe kidneys must be imaged preoperatively by CT-KUB at minimum, preferably a CT-IVP to avoid potential bowel injury, ascertain the depth from the skin to the outermost calyx and identify the location and size of the calculi.

Chapter 2
Personnel and Equipment

This chapter lists the equipment that I prefer for PCNL, i.e. what works for me. All manufacturers produce excellent instruments. All personnel, nurses, theatre technicians, surgeons and assistants, must have previous PCNL experience and training.

Medical Personnel

- Anaesthetist:
  The anaesthetist must be familiar with PCNL. Specific experience is required for positioning the head and airway (prone, face support and protection, renal bolster, airway management).
  – Patient position: prone, "swimming position" of arms, I.V. line in the forward arm on the side of the stone.
  – Bairhugger and temperature control.
  – "TUR syndrome".
  – Cessation of respiration in inspiration for needle puncture.
  – Awareness of potential problems and appreciation of the need to alert the surgeon early, i.e. blood loss, hypotension, hypothermia and "TUR syndrome".
  – Awareness of possible pneumothorax with supra costal approaches.
  – Potential for air embolism with retrograde air injection during the renal puncture.
- Nursing:
  – Experienced PCNL nurses:
    PCNL is technical and complex. Endoscopes, lithotrites, guide wires, graspers and nephrostomies are all procedure specific. The theatre nurse must have the ability to anticipate surgical requirements, and have all the equipment tested and functional before the skin puncture is made. The surgeon cannot

interrupt a difficult procedure to wait for faulty or unchecked equipment, e.g. sonotrode malfunction.
- Theatre technician/orderly:
PCNL requires uninterrupted function of the light source, monitors, suction, sonotrode, pneumatic lithotripter and fluid irrigation. Any breakdown can be critical. Patient positioning and transfer are also critical.
- Radiographer:
The radiographer must be familiar with PCNL, placement of the C-arm, collimation or coning, parallax, and have a good rapport and communication with the surgeon. It is important that the surgeon gives precise requests to the radiographer, which they both understand, e.g. "snapshot", "continuous screen", "rotate the C-arm on its axis" and so on.
- Assistant:
Must understand the principals of radiation, the nature of percutaneous surgery and the critical responsibility of maintaining the guide wire in the kidney. Junior residents should not be allowed to assist at PCNL without previous observation and instruction. Having a guide wire displaced as a result of assistant inexperience is stressful and potentially disastrous.
- Surgeon:
The surgeon is entirely dependent on the theatre team. The surgeon cannot control the imaging, set up or maintain the technical equipment. Rapport between the surgeon and the entire theatre team is paramount.

Equipment Requirements

Operation Table

Requirements

- Lithotomy and screening.
- Eccentric operating table columns to enable the C-arm to be positioned below the patient to screen from the bladder to the kidney.
- Arm boards in the "swimming" position.

Patient Positioning

Requirements

- Multiple pillows.
- Covered sponge triangular renal bolsters and flat pads for the kidney, hips and chest.

- "Trauma beanbag" (for spinal cord injury patients and patients with skeletal deformities, e.g. spina bifida).
- Patient trolley (to roll the patient on and off the operating table during the transfer from lithotomy).

Imaging

- X-ray display box or digital monitor. All preoperative x-ray images must be available and on display before the procedure commences.
- The images should be clearly visible to the surgeon for reference during the procedure.

C-ARM

- Access requirements
- Lithotomy
  For retrograde catheter, ureteric stone manipulation and insertion of stent if required.

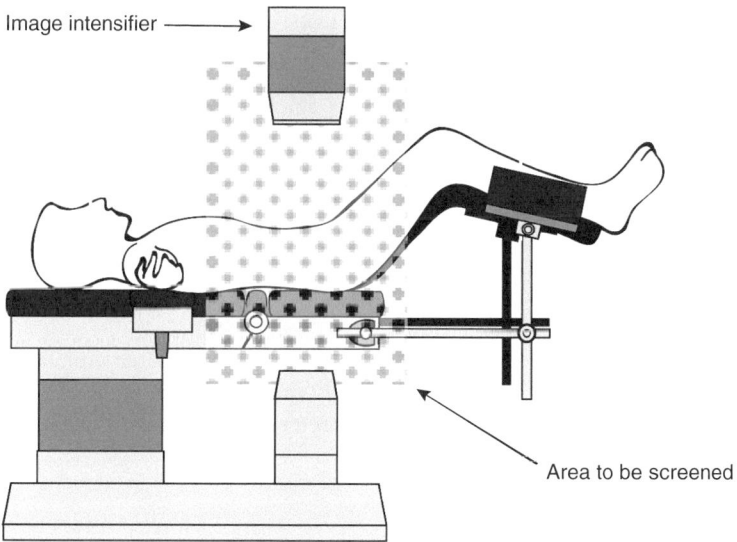

Fig. 2.1 Area to be imaged during radiological screening in lithotomy

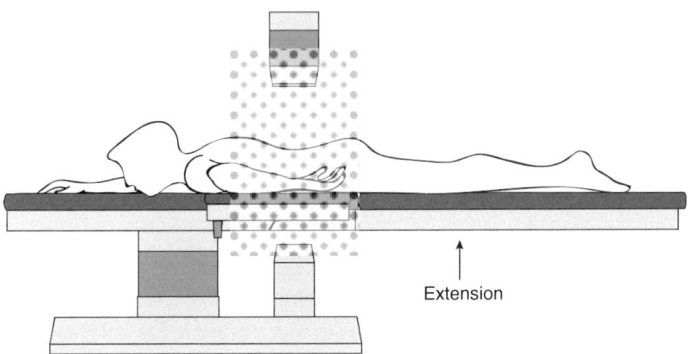

Fig. 2.2 Area to be screened for PCNL in the prone position

- PCNL
  Must have free access from the lower chest to the bladder and be able to rotate the C-arm from side to side for parallax II screening during the renal puncture.

Access

The surgeon must control the imaging of the upper urinary tract. This requires a 5–6 Fr retrograde ureteric catheter (RGC) inserted cystoscopically to lie within the renal pelvis. If the catheter tip is below the PUJ, it can be very difficult or impossible to image and dilate all the calyces for puncture. The RGC must be fixed to a urethral catheter by adhesive tape to prevent displacement.

Retrograde contrast should be a "50–50" solution of saline and contrast medium with a few drops only of methylene blue. The surgeon requires direct access to the external tip of the RGC to inject contrast, saline with methylene blue, insert guide wires and to establish a "universal guide wire" (UGW).

Hydrophilic or "Slippery" Guide Wires

These are my preference. They do not kink. They can be held atraumatically with artery forceps. They flex, coil and pass easily into the pelvis without trauma and are particularly useful when negotiating ureteric stones. They are essential if using the single-stage dilator because they do not kink. The cystoscopic guide wire can be reused for the renal puncture following the insertion of the retrograde catheter.

"Slippery" wires are more expensive than standard metal guide wires. Due to their springiness and lack of friction, "slippery wires" can "flip out" of the collecting system, especially if put in the hands of an inexperienced assistant!

Artery Forceps

Artery forceps are used to hold guide wires, dilate the lumbodorsal fascia and act as skin markers for the needle puncture. I prefer straight artery forceps because they need to pass parallel to the guide wire when dilating the lumbodorsal fascia.

Retrograde Catheter

I use a 6 Fr gauge open-ended RGC with a Leur lock proximally.
Open-ended catheters are necessary

- To pass over a guide wire
- For flushing calculi in the ureter
- To establish a universal guide wire

Urethral Catheter

16 Fr Foley

Functions
- Drain bladder.
- Attach and fix retrograde catheter tape. I prefer one-inch waterproof tape, known commercially as "Sleek". The tape should be "suitably fashioned", i.e. the ends folded over so that the assistant can detach the tape under the drapes if required, with a "mesentery" to properly fix the ureteric catheter to the urethral catheter.

Fixation of the Ureteric Catheter Prior to Placing the Patient Prone

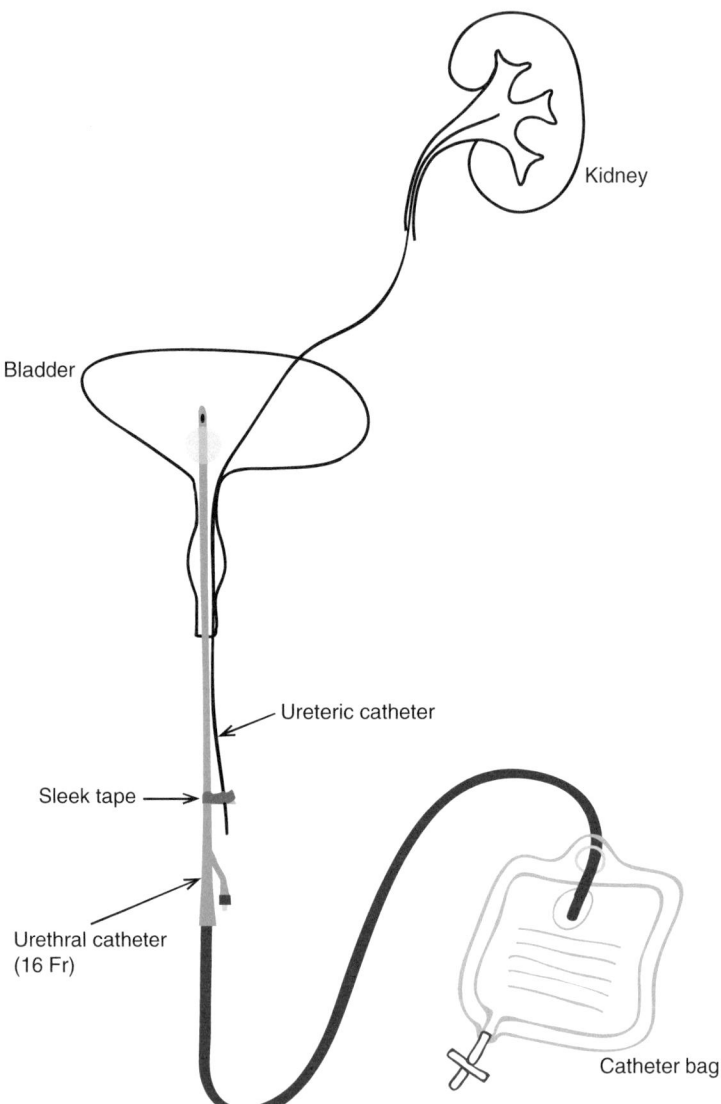

Fig. 2.3 Urinary catheters and drainage for PCNL

Fig. 2.4 Method of attaching the ureteric catheter to the Foley Catheter so that it can be easily accessed and will not slip during PCNL

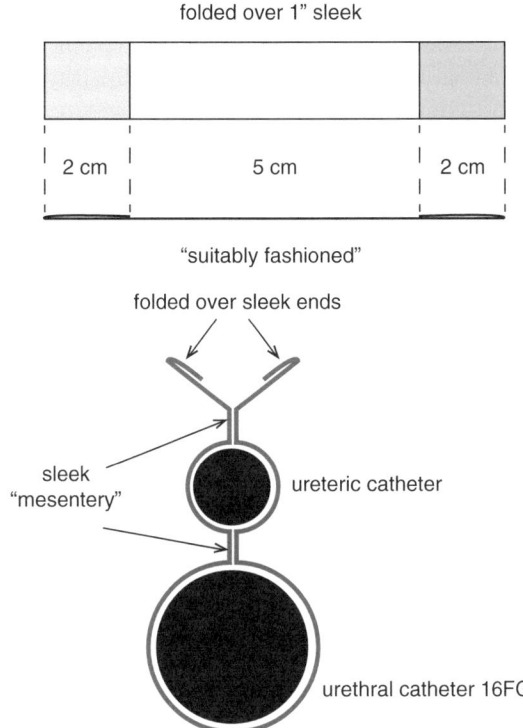

Contrast

We use Urograffin 70 % 50 ml mixed with 50 ml 0.9 % saline and 0.5 ml of methylene blue, just enough to give the injected contrast mixture a faint blue tinge. The methylene blue concentration should be just light enough to distinguish aspirated contrast from urine, but not so dark as to confuse the aspirate with blood.

Contrast should not be infused at the time of retrograde catheter insertion when the patient is in lithotomy, except in particular circumstances such as identifying the pelviureteric junction when performing an endoscopic pyeloplasty, when dealing with a radiolucent calculus or to delineate ureteric anatomy, such as with bifid ureter. Retrograde contrast infusion is also indicated where there is a suggestion that there has been a ureteric injury, or the guide wire cannot be manipulated into the kidney. In a routine PCNL for stone, infusion of contrast prior to screening for the renal puncture will mask the location of the stone. Minimum volume extension tubing (140 cm, Pkt 25) is attached to the 6 Fr RGC proximal Leur lock after positioning the patient for the PCNL to enable the surgeon to infuse contrast for the renal puncture. With this arrangement, the surgeon can inject the contrast.

Patient Drape

Once prone, the drape must attach to the patient, be waterproof and have an access window for the puncture and nephrostomy access. We find that craniofacial neurosurgical drapes are ideal, and use the barrier Craniotomy Drape (Ref. 888442) by Molnlycke Health Care.

Bairhugger: Blankets and Drapes

Patients can rapidly develop hypothermia due to convection from the spread of fluid over the body surface, so drapes must be waterproof. Heat reflective "Space Blankets", plastic sheeting or a second Bairhugger (depending on availability) should be used below the level of the urethral catheter to maintain temperature and dryness over the lower extremities. A warming Bairhugger is preferable for the upper chest, shoulders and arms.

These precautions are particularly critical during paediatric PCNL, where the effects of blood loss and cooling are magnified.

Antibiotics

All patients are given antibiotics with the induction of anaesthesia whether their urine cultures are positive or sterile. Patients with obstructive calculi, particularly those with neurogenic bladders or urinary diversions may be admitted 48 h prior to surgery for nephrostomy and parenteral antibiotics. Our routine prophylaxis is a cephalosporin and aminoglycoside.

DVT: Prophylaxis

Although DVT is uncommon following PCNL, we fit all our patients with below-knee thromboembolism-deterrent stockings prior to PCNL. In high-risk patients, we use Clexane and pneumatic calf compressors.

Scalpel

A sharp-pointed no. 11 or no. 15 scalpel blade is required to make a small stab through the dermis before inserting the PCNL needle.

Guide Wires

We routinely use the Terumo 0.035 inch × 100 cm "slippery" hydrophilic guide wire with a straight floppy tip. These are atraumatic, coil easily in the kidney, readily "find their way" along the ureter and bypass calculi.

However, they are springy and can easily "flip out" of the kidney and can slip through the surgeon's fingers. We always hold these slippery wires with artery forceps.

Also, as these wires are straight tipped, they may pass through and out of the collecting system during a "through and through" puncture, and may also be difficult to advance between the stone and collecting system where the stone is tightly impacted. In these situations, we use a "J-wire" (where the tip is a half circle). We routinely keep an unopened "J-wire" on the urology trolley. The 'J-wire' comes with an introducer ("golf tee") which straightens the tip so the wire can be introduced into the PCN cannula.

Guide Wires-Types

- "Slippery" guide wire
- Metal
- Straight wire with floppy "J" tip
- Super stiff guide wire with floppy tip

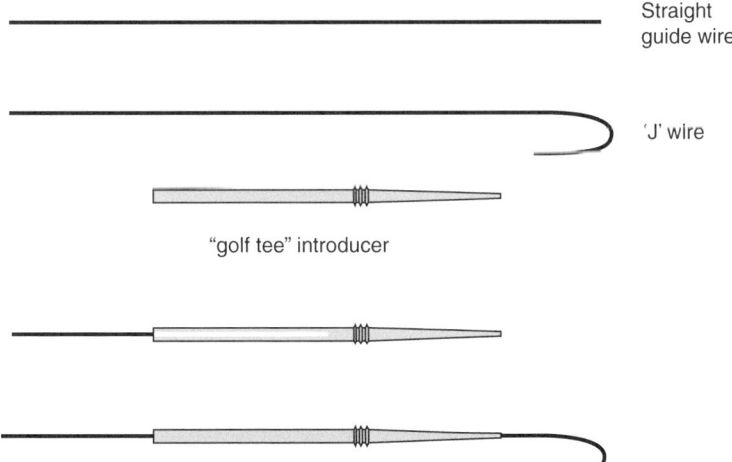

Fig. 2.5 Guide wires and the "Golf Tee" introducer

Nephrostomy Track Dilators

Five Varieties

- Amplatz serial exchange dilators
- Metal telescoping dilators ("car aerial")
- Balloon dilators
- Webb single-stage dilator
- "Mini Perc" single-stage dilators

Characteristics of Various Dilators

Amplatz Serial Exchange Dilators

Positives

- Familiar
- Smooth
- Flexible
- Tapered tip
- Often the best dilator in the presence of dense scar tissue

Negatives

- Long and cumbersome internal 8 Fr "guide" or "long grey" inner dilator.
- Single use.
- The entire set has to be opened (expensive) even if only using one dilator.
- Bleeding occurs between dilator exchanges.
- For a large hydronephrosis, the kidney can collapse and fall off the dilators between dilators exchanges.
- Serial exchanges takes time.
- With serial exchanges, the guide wire can be easily displaced, particularly if it is not well anchored within the kidney (such as within a calyceal diverticulum)
- The Amplatz system is a three-stage procedure requiring arterial dilators to commence the track before placing the "long grey" and subsequent Amplatz dilators.
- The Amplatz dilator's leading nose is blunt and can displace the kidney.

Telescopic "Car Aerial" Dilators (Alken)

Positives

- Cheap
- Reusable forever (single purchase)
- Do not deflate a hydronephrotic system as there is no serial exchange
- Tamponade the parenchyma, preventing bleeding between each dilator insertion
- Autoclavable (metal)

Guide Wires

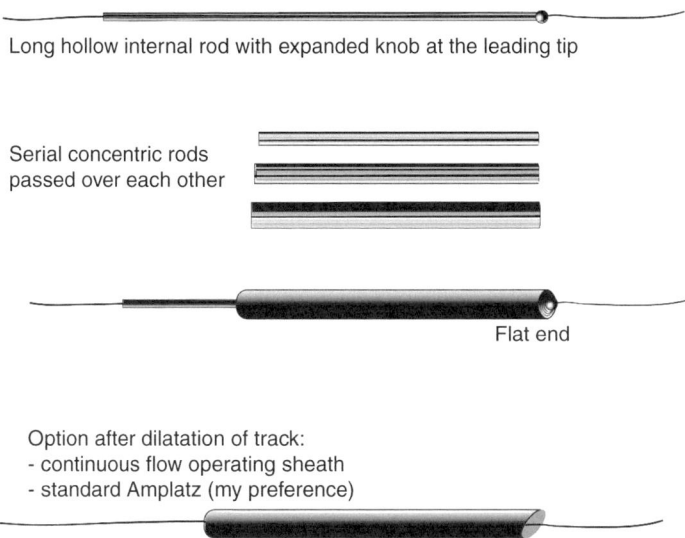

Fig. 2.6 The Alken "car aerial" dilator system

Negatives

- Flat internal distal end of stacked dilators can displace the kidney and the calculus.
- Long 8 Fr central rod (60 cm) can be cumbersome.
- Difficult to insert in the presence of a rigid curved track.
- It can be difficult with II imaging to accurately see the end of the advancing dilator.
- Can be difficult to pass the dilators through dense scar tissue.

Balloon Dilators

Operative Procedure

1. Renal puncture and insertion of guide wire
2. Fascial dilator over guide wire
3. Balloon inserted over the guide wire into the kidney
4. Balloon inflated
5. Large dilator over balloon (not in all makes)
6. Amplatz sheath over last dilator or balloon

Positives

- Tamponades the kidney during inflation of the balloon.

Negatives

- Expensive.
- Single use (disposable).

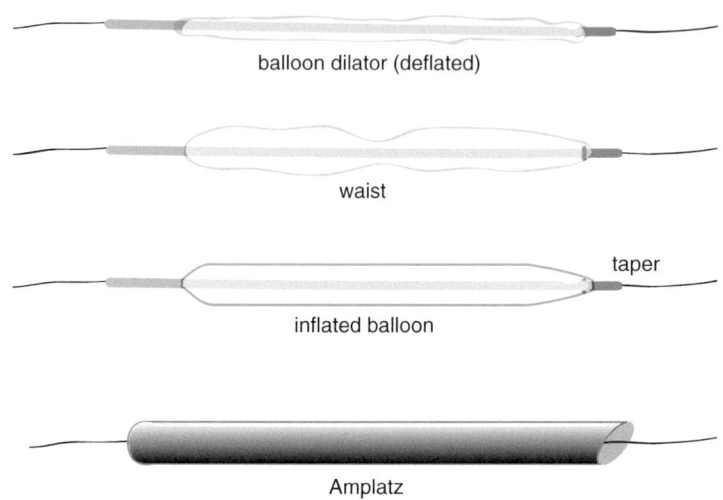

Fig. 2.7 Balloon dilator system

- May require up to three dilations (depending on the brand) before the final Amplatz sheath is inserted. During these exchanges, the initial tamponade can be lost.
- The balloon can "waist" in the body, particularly where it passes through scar tissue or traversing the lumbodorsal fascia.
- The leading edge of the balloon tip is tapered, so it may extrude during inflation (especially in a very confined space such as a calyceal diverticulum or staghorn calculus).
- Scar tissue – may be too rigid for the balloon to expand.

Webb Single-Stage Dilator

This system employs only one dilator and one Amplatz sheath, which are inserted over the nephrostomy guide wire as a single manoeuvre.

Technique of Insertion

Positives

- Cheap (single dilator and Amplatz sheath combined).
- Disposable.
- Tamponades track during introduction as only a single dilatation.

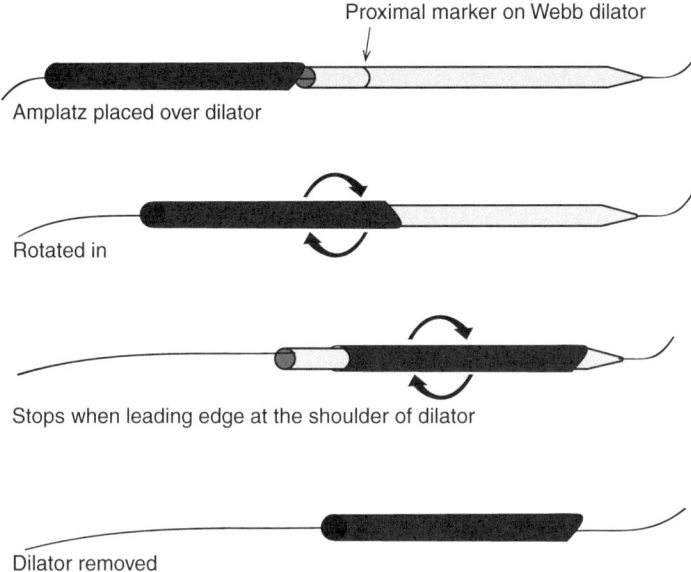

Fig. 2.8 Webb single-stage dilator system

- Will not deflate a hydronephrotic collecting system.
- Fast (single-stage) dilatation.
- Do not require a large area of intrarenal space.
- Simple single insertion of the dilator.
- Screening is not required during the insertion of the Amplatz sheath, as the depth is marked by a proximal line on the dilator.
- Will not cause pneumothorax when passing through pleura because there is no dilator exchange and the dilator is removed after Amplatz sheath has been introduced into the kidney.

Negatives

- Can displace the kidney if the kidney is very mobile
- Requires a hydrophilic guide wire and experience

"Mini Perc" Dilators

These are metal single-stage dilators. They share the same characteristics as the Webb dilator, are reusable and autoclavable. The two larger dilators for the 16.5/19.5 Fr and 21/24 Fr sheaths have a double lumen, allowing the surgeon to insert a safety wire as well as an operative wire with the first passage of the dilator.

Alternative techniques of SSD

It is possible to perform a one (or two) dilator SSD access track using a 24Fr or 26Fr Cook Amplatz dilator directly over the long hollow internal rod of the Alken car aerial set or the 8Fr "long grey" inner dilator of the Cook Amplatz Renal Dilator Set..

Amplatz Sheath

The Amplatz sheath is a firm circular Teflon or polyurethane tube.

The Amplatz sheath is an open-ended sheath which provides a conduit for endoscopic access from the skin into the renal collecting system.

The inner surface of the sheath is applied intimately to the dilator.

The leading edge of the Amplatz sheath is obliquely offset and so is oval in cross section. This leading edge is bevelled and sharp, and may cut tissues if the sheath is introduced into the kidney when not firmly applied to the dilator, or if the sheath advances further than the shoulder of the dilator, or it is advanced blindly in the absence of a dilator.

Advantages

- The Amplatz sheath enables free flow of irrigant, stone particles and blood in and out of the kidney.
- The Amplatz sheath allows easy and safe insertion of a nephrostomy.
- Being an open-ended conduit, it is not possible to create a high pressure perfusion of the kidney, as no matter what height the irrigant flows from, the hydrostatic

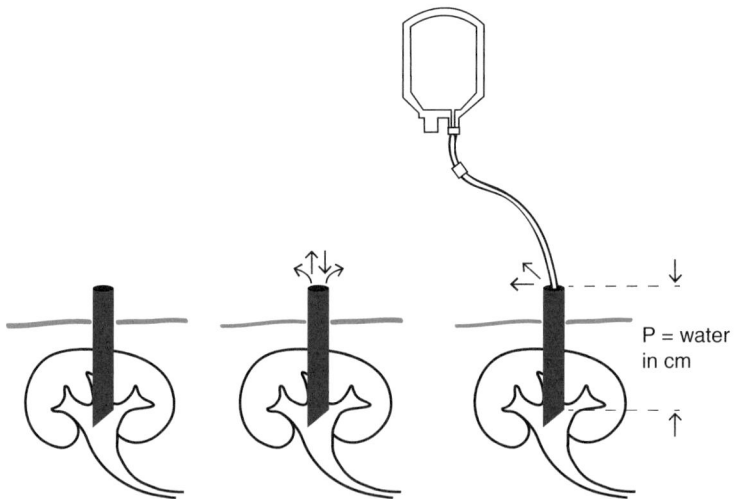

Fig. 2.9 Hydrostatic pressure of irrigant in the open system Amplatz sheath

pressure within the kidney is always equal the height of the outer end of the Amplatz sheath above the kidney in centimetres of water, so the operating irrigant hydrostatic pressure is always less than 10 cm of water (see Fig. 2.9).
- The Amplatz sheath is versatile.
- It may be split and extracted around a nephrostomy tube (peel away technique).

The "peel away" sheath is created by the surgeon, dividing the outer sheath with heavy scissors by two parallel incisions directly opposite each other.

To remove the sheath, the two outer flaps created by the incisions are grasped by artery forceps. By slowly pulling these artery forceps apart, the sheath splits into two and can be gently extracted without disturbing the kidney or nephrostomy.

- An Amplatz sheath can be extended to create a long access conduit for use for PCNL in long body wall tracks such as in obesity or horseshoe kidney.

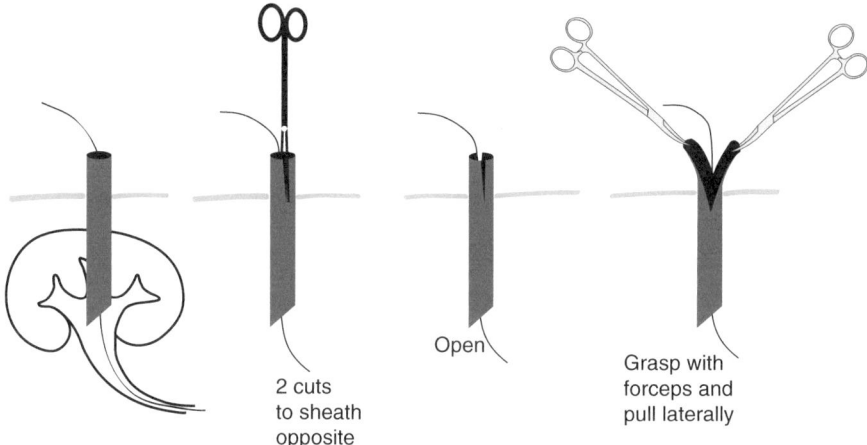

Fig. 2.10 Technique of creating a "peel away" Amplatz sheath

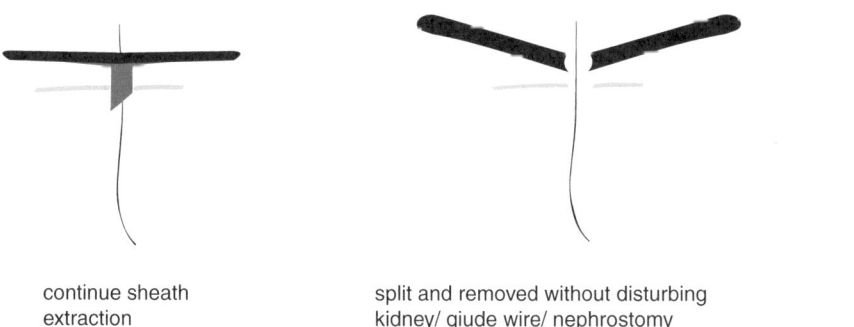

Fig. 2.11 Final steps in "peel away" sheath removal

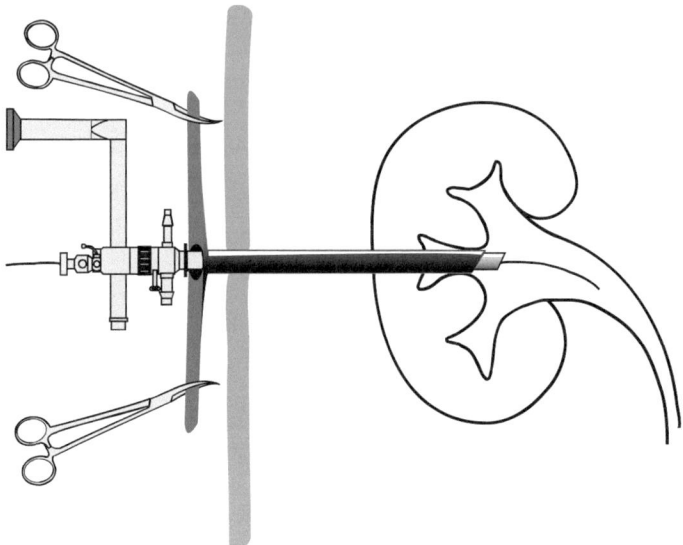

Fig. 2.12 Creation of a "short" Amplatz sheath

In situations where the nephroscope tip is deep in the kidney, such as entering the upper ureter, the surgeon may inadvertently advance the Amplatz sheath as a result of the proximal hub of the nephroscope pushing on the outer end of the sheath. As the leading or internal end of the Amplatz is proximal to the surgeon's view, the sheath can cut and damage the collecting system. This can be avoided by splitting the sheath down to the skin externally, as for the "peel away" removal technique, allowing further excursion of the nephroscope into the kidney without inadvertent sheath advancement.

Considerations When Using the Amplatz Sheath System

Sheath Size Selection

French gauge (Fr) is the circumference of the instrument in millimetres. It is natural to assume the diameter of the instrument to be a third of the Fr. However, many endoscopic instruments are oval in shape. As a result, their maximum diameter is wider than their French gauge sizing (i.e. implied diameter) would imply. Therefore, most instruments require a larger Amplatz sheath than their quoted French size would suggest. The surgeon should test the nephroscope in the intended Amplatz sheath before commencing track dilation.

Fig. 2.13 Comparison of the Fr (French gauge) of a circular sheath and an oval instrument

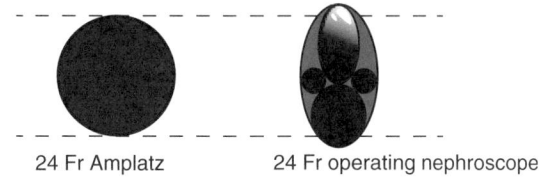

24 Fr Amplatz   24 Fr operating nephroscope

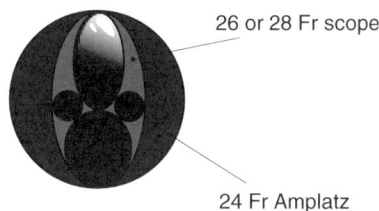

26 or 28 Fr scope

24 Fr Amplatz

Test before commence dilation

Avoiding Trauma from the Amplatz Sheath

- Only advance the sheath over a correctly sized dilator.
- Always monitor the advancing dilator by II, ensuring the leading edge of the sheath does not go past the shoulder of the tip of the dilator.
- When using a Webb dilator, ensure that the external end of the Amplatz sheath does not go deeper than the external safety marker on the shaft of the Webb dilator.
- Never advance an Amplatz sheath blindly.
- Only ever advance the Amplatz sheath over a dilator, unless under vision in a large capacious renal pelvis or calyx.
- Only ever advance the sheath without a dilator under vision when the collecting system and all the inner edge of the Amplatz sheath are visible.

Puncture Needle

Features

- Purpose built
- Length is 1–2 cm longer than the Amplatz sheath.
- Stiff and springy, so it will create a straight track through the body wall.
- We prefer an oblique bevelled tip rather than a tapered diamond tip.

- Utilising the angle of the bevel, the surgeon can manipulate the tip of the needle to create a curve in the track.
- The angle of the bevel is identified by a mark on the external Leur lock of the needle, to enable the surgeon to identify the bevel direction internally.
- Transparent sheath – the surgeon can confirm entry to the collection system by the appearance of methylene blue coloured contrast either spontaneously or with a very small aspiration.
- Often a faint tinge of blood in the aspirate obscures the methylene blue, so it is not clear if one is aspirating urine or contrast. In this situation, ask the radiographer to take a "snapshot" picture. If contrast is in the sheath, it will show on the image. We call this the "STREAK" sign.
- The length of the needle is sufficient to create a "Y" puncture through the Amplatz sheath.

Irrigation Fluid

Irrigation fluid must be isotonic and warm. We use normal saline (Baxter 0.9 % Sodium Chloride, 2 l bags) routinely and Glycine if diathermy is anticipated, e.g. for transitional cell ablation. The 2 l bags are suspended on a separate IV pole using a "Y" or dual-chamber giving set. Both bags are open, with one placed higher than the other, to avoid loss of irrigation during the procedure.

The bags are about 60–80 cm above the patient. Height is not crucial when using the Amplatz sheath as the system is open, preventing excessive hydrostatic pressure.

Nephroscopes

- Rigid
- Flexible

The majority are rigid.

The lens eyepiece is offset to enable the passage of rigid instruments (lithotrites/graspers, etc.).

The lens may be a right angle 90° "crank handle" configuration or at a 30° offset from the shaft.

The development of these two configurations is historical, related to pre video monitor days when the surgeon's face, when looking directly into the eyepiece, would often clash with the patient's buttock when using a 90° nephroscope, known at the time as the "cheek to cheek syndrome"!

The choice of nephroscope is a personal preference. Rigid endoscopes have excellent vision (rod lens fibre optic), irrigation and working channels. Being rigid, their manoeuvrability through long tracks (e.g. horseshoe kidneys) or around complex intrarenal anatomy is limited by distance and the spatial location of calculi in the calyces.

Flexible endoscopes are less hardy and more expensive than rigid nephroscopes.

Their flexibility limits instrumentation to flexible instruments and stone fragmentation by laser lithotripsy.

Flexible nephroscopes are particularly useful for long, complex tracks such as those in horseshoe kidneys or obese patients.

They are also excellent for "second look" nephroscopies under local anaesthesia and sedation following a previous formal PCNL – e.g. staghorn calculi.

Instruments for Intracorporal Stone Fragmentation

The two commonly used lithotrites are the solid rod metal pneumatic probes (e.g. lithoclast) and the metal hollow vibrating and aspirating ultrasonic lithotrite. The "ultrasound" probe fragments the stone by vibrations generated by a piezoelectric crystal proximally.

The pneumatic pulses and piezoelectric 'ultrasound' generated vibrations break stones by a "jack hammer" effect.

Unless using a flexible nephroscope or fragmenting small calculi (e.g. "mini perc" or paediatric PCNL), I tend not to use laser fragmentation which is less effective within the kidney than the ureter.

Laser fibres are fine and expensive. However, they can be useful in confined spaces for "stone dusting".

Electro-hydraulic probes used during the early development of PCNL have been superseded by the ultrasonic and pneumatic lithoclasts.

Electro-hydraulic probes can damage mucosa and telescopes if used incorrectly.

Pneumatic Ballistic Lithotrites (Lithoclast)

Indications

- Large, hard, heavily calcified calculi
- Large struvite calculi, particularly within the renal pelvis, where there is space around the stone
- Large calcified cysteine or urate calculi
- Very hard calculi, e.g. apatite
- Smaller ureteric calculi
- Small renal and calyceal calculi (Mini-Perc)

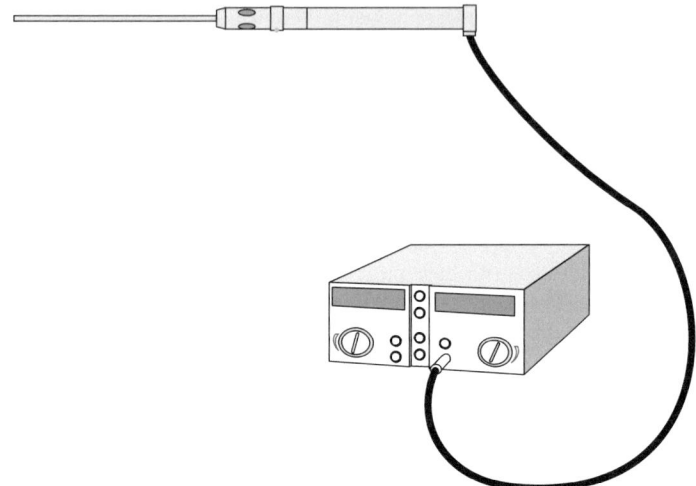

Fig. 2.14 The pneumatic lithoclast

Advantages

- Hardy.
- Can break all stones, especially very hard dense calculi.
- Simple and cheap with minimal ongoing costs.
- Driven by compressed air.
- Reusable.
- Probes never wear out.
- Frequency and pressure can be adjusted to perform large stone fragmentation or fine "stone dusting".

Disadvantages

- The probe cannot remove or aspirate calculi. When used in a confined space, the surgeon must re-enter the kidney repeatedly with the nephroscope. This can result in bleeding, loss of track, clot formation and stone fragment displacement.
- When used in the ureter, the probe can retropulse and displace stones proximally along the lumen.
- Stones require immobilisation for the probe to be effective. This may be difficult in a large renal pelvis.
- Prolonged use of the lithoclast in a confined space may cause bleeding.

Sonotrode

Advantages

- Excellent and rapid fragmentation of soft calculi, e.g. struvite stones.
- Aspirates particles, so very useful in confined spaces such as the ureter, calyceal diverticula, or stones impacted within calyces. The sonotrode can remove large

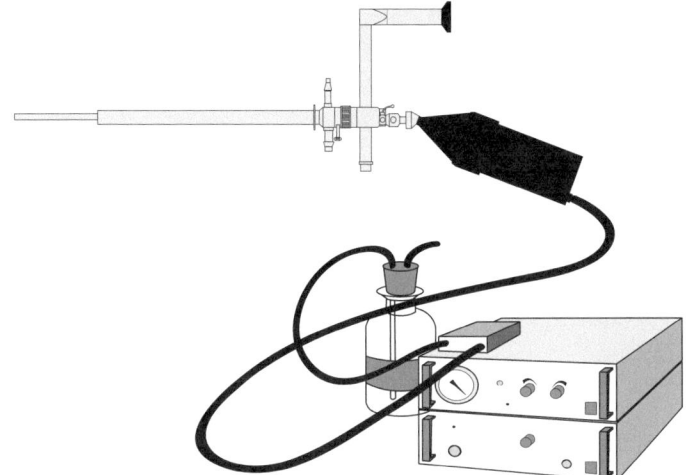

Fig. 2.15 Hollow-probe ultrasound lithotrite with generator box and suction pump

volumes of stone without needing to remove and re-insert the nephroscope, avoiding track loss and bleeding.
- Aspiration assists with keeping the visual field clear during bleeding.
- Atraumatic to tissues.
- Small stone fragments that are difficult to grasp can be aspirated.

Disadvantages

- Set up is complicated and requires an experienced technician (particularly the suction pump and tubing).
- Does not break hard calculi well.
- Continuous aspiration can collapse the collecting system of the kidney, limiting vision and irrigation.
- Probes overheat very quickly if irrigation ceases, which may cause thermal damage to the patient, surgeon, and burn out the piezoelectric generator.
- Replacement probes are expensive.
- The probes are hollow and so relatively large, so they do not "miniaturize" sufficiently for "mini-PCNL" or fine ureteroscopy.
- The sonotrode must be applied directly onto the stone with varying degrees of pressure to break a calculus, so the stone must be immobilised.
- This pressure may displace stone fragments, physically damage the collecting system, and even push stone fragments out through the collecting system.

Equipment for Percutaneous Endoscopic Pyloplasty (or Endopyelotomy)

- Storz visual urethrotome sheath
- Zero degree cystoscope lens

- Working element (TUR)
- Back cutting "sickle knife" (Storz)
- Two straight, "slippery" guide wires

Stone Grasping Instruments

Graspers

Alligator Forceps

These have a "scissor handle", which manoeuvres the distally hinged jaws.

The jaws are small and open outwards in a "V". They have a small, relatively fragile hinge and a blunt distal nose. The jaws clamp onto stone fragments in a forward action. As a result, the alligator forceps cannot grasp large fragments, as attempting to engage fragments of stone will push them away as the jaws close.

The jaws of the alligator forceps are ribbed, and they are very effective at removing small stone fragments, 4 mm or less.

The jaws are narrow and so do not grasp or extract clots effectively.

As the jaws are hinged and the proximal handles are strong, grasping large stones will break the hinge (which is expensive!).

Due to the hinge, the alligator forceps jaws can open in small spaces, even within the ureter, as neither the shaft of the instrument nor the nephroscope have to be retracted to enable the jaws to open.

As the tips of the jaws are smooth, they can be inserted into renal parenchyma and opened under vision, to atraumatically separate the parenchyma and so create an atraumatic nephrostomy track (very useful when the renal dilator cannot be fully inserted into a calyx, e.g. staghorn calculus, calyceal diverticulum).

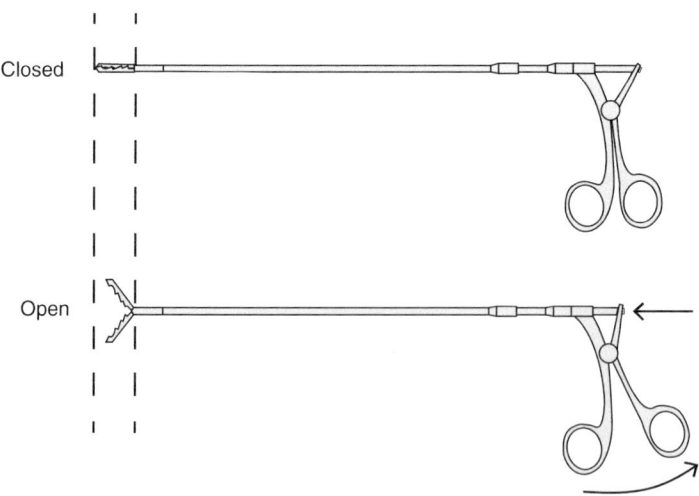

Fig. 2.16 Alligator forceps open and close without needing to withdraw the forceps

Stone Grasping Instruments

Triradiate Forceps

These have a simple mechanism without joints or hinges. They are easily sterilised, and are cheap and strong.

Stones are grasped by sharp-pointed tines, which have a backwards-facing sharp single claw at the tip. The tips of the tines spread out widely, entrap the stone, and grasp it by retracting backwards towards the instrument, the clawed tips holding the stone.

The triradiate tines can hold larger stone fragments than alligator forceps.

The tines are sharp. They can easily perforate the collecting system, and may tear and lacerate the kidney or collecting system during closure, due to the sharp backwards-facing claws.

To embrace and grasp a calculus, the tines must pass the stone for up to a centimetre. If that is not possible (e.g. when the stone is against the wall of the pelvis) then the shaft of the triradiate grasper must be retracted, and as a result, so does the nephroscope. Therefore, the safe deployment of the triradiate grasper is restricted to stones in larger open spaces.

In practice, triradiate forceps have limited use in confined spaces where they cannot embrace the stone, such as in a calyx. The triradiate forceps can be dangerous in the ureter, as the tines, when advancing to grasp the stone, can easily perforate the ureteric wall and closure of the tines result in the claws, lacerating the ureter like a fish-hook.

The triradiate tines do not oppose to each other as effectively as alligator forceps, so they are inefficient for removing small fragments. Small stone particles (<4 mm) slip between the tines.

As with alligator forceps, triradiate forceps are poor at extracting clots.

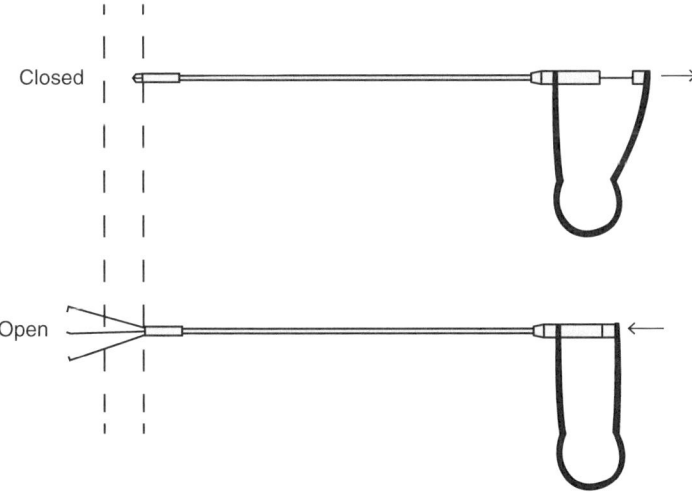

Fig. 2.17 Triradiate forceps demonstrating the forward excursion required to open the tines

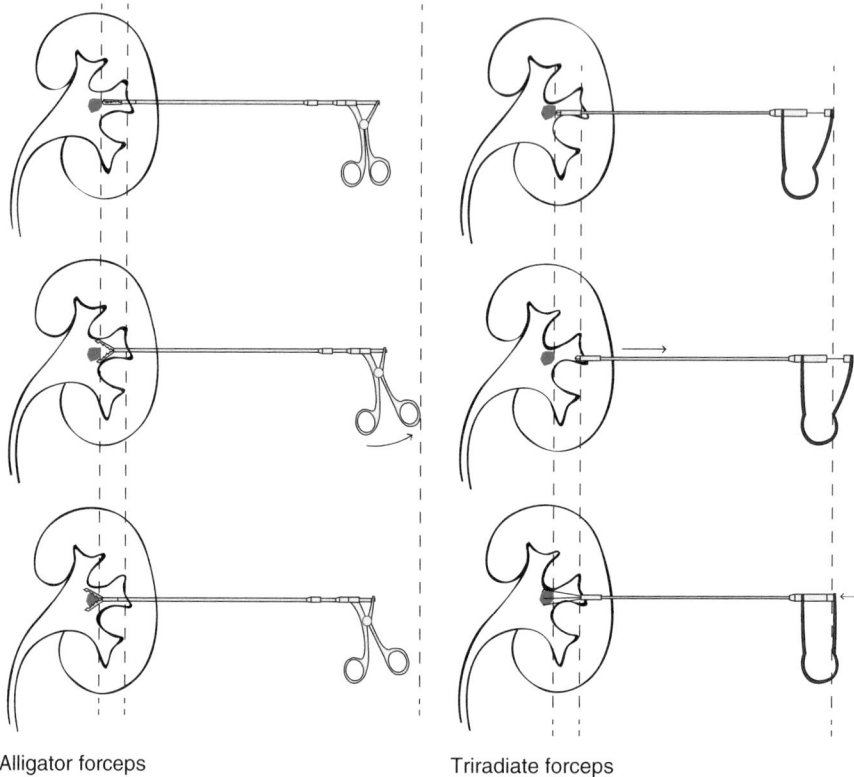

Fig. 2.18 Comparison of alligator and triradiate forceps. The triradiate forceps have to be retracted to grasp a stone; the alligator forceps do not

Nephrostomies

Most urologists leave a nephrostomy in the kidney following PCNL to drain the kidney primarily of urine, (blood drains poorly through any nephrostomy) to allow further imaging such as a nephrostoureterogram, and provide a route for re-entry to the kidney. A nephrostomy provides a low-pressure vent, allowing any collecting system trauma to resolve. We do not believe that a large nephrostomy provides better drainage or tamponade. Small (10–14 Fr) Cope nephrostomies drain urine well and allow the nephrostomy track to "collapse" to its normal anatomy. Low-grade and venous bleeding settles by tamponade and clotting. Significant arterial bleeding resists even balloon tamponade and requires radiological embolisation.

If the kidney is bleeding, we believe a nephrostomy provides better drainage than a stent.

Nephrostomy Types

- Loop (Cope)

Stone Grasping Instruments

- Balloon catheters
- Malecot
- "Tubeless", i.e. double J stent

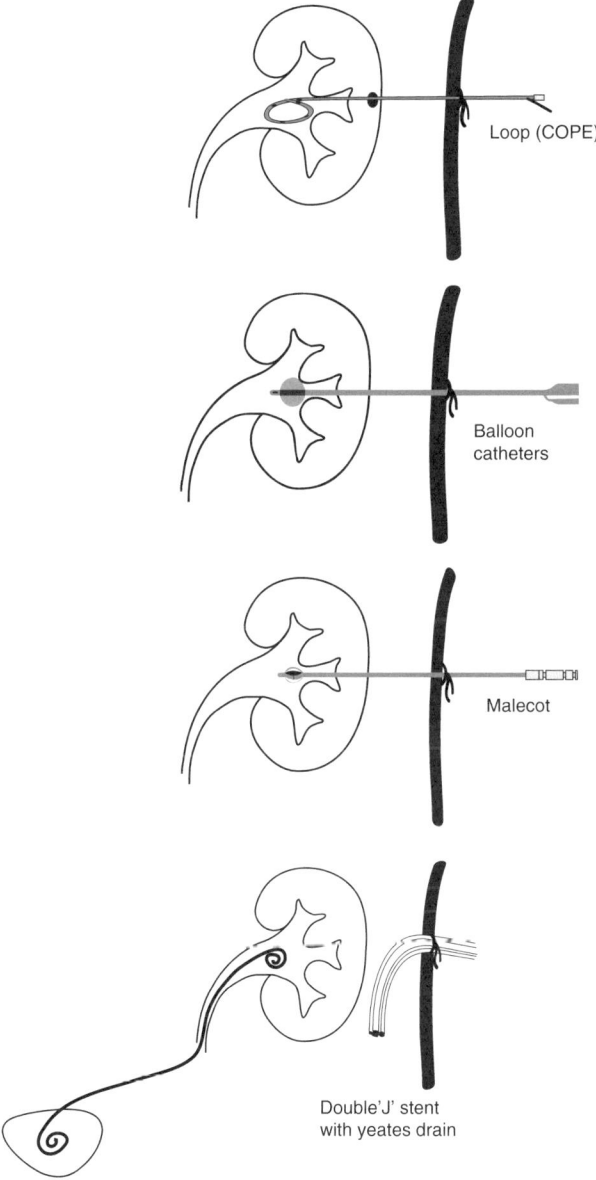

Fig. 2.19 The Cope loop, Foley balloon, Malecot catheter and double J stent or "tubeless" nephrostomies

Cope Nephrostomy

These are a simple fine tube self-retaining nephrostomy with an internal string to form a retaining loop inside the kidney.

Advantages

- Cheap.
- Can be used for nephrostogram or reinsertion of a guide wire.
- Easily removed on the ward.
- Give excellent access for a radiologist should a second procedure be required such an antegrade insertion of stent or antegrade basket extraction.
- Are soft and flexible, allowing free movement with respiration and patient comfort.

Disadvantages

- It can be difficult to shape the loop within the kidney, particularly in a small collecting system, e.g. calyceal diverticulum.
- Ward staff require education on how to safely release the internal string maintaining the Cope loop. Otherwise, should the loop not release and straighten, removal of the nephrostomy can cause pain, tearing or trauma to the parenchyma and bleeding from the kidney.
- The string and loop of the Cope nephrostomy can become tangled with the upper end of a double J stent, and inadvertently extract the double J stent with nephrostomy removal.
- Surgeons must be aware of this potential complication. If a Cope nephrostomy and double J stent coexist, the Cope nephrostomy must be removed over a guide wire under II control in the radiology department to prevent displacement of the ureteric stent by nephrostomy removal.

Foley Balloon Catheters

- While these are readily available and commonly used, I do not favour them. The balloon can be difficult or impossible to deflate and their subsequent removal difficult.
- The catheters are rigid and so can be uncomfortable with respiration.
- A Foley catheter only drains via a hole at the tip of the catheter and this opening can become obstructed in the small renal collecting system.

Other Drain Tubes

It is sometimes impossible to insert a nephrostomy tube into the kidney; the track may be lost before inserting a nephrostomy. In this situation, it is a simple matter for the surgeon to place a Penrose drain, a round drain tube or a Yeates drain along the nephrostomy track next to the kidney (similar to open renal surgery).

Some urologists also insert a double J stent in this circumstance. I rarely do and only if the procedure has been long or complicated.

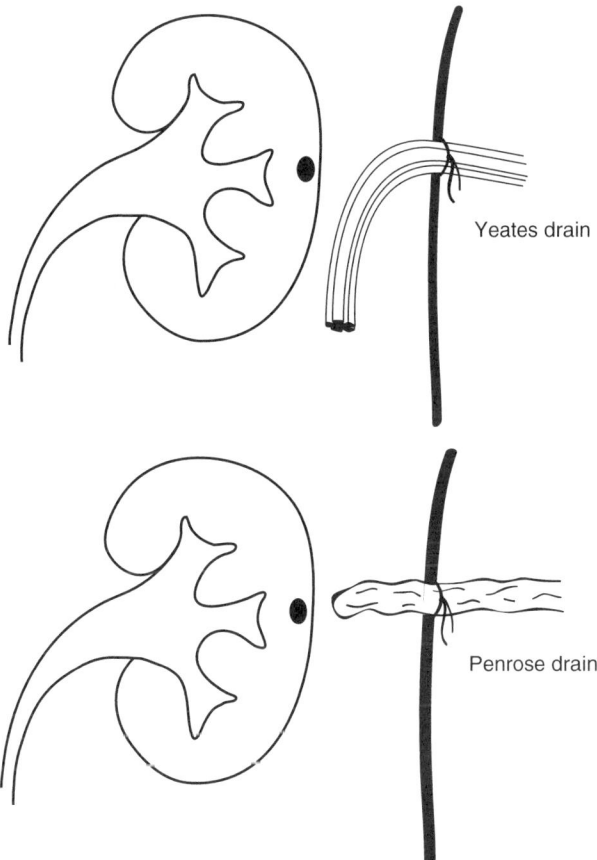

Fig. 2.20 Simple perirenal drain tubes without nephrostomy

Tubeless Nephrostomy

In a straightforward nephrolithotomy or endoscopic pyeloplasty, or where the PCNL has traversed the pleura, it is common practice to insert an internal Double J stent only and no external nephrostomy, the so-called "tubeless" nephrostomy.

Chest Drains

In the case of a significant pneumothorax, a formal chest drain may be required.

Chapter 3
Indications for PCNL

Introduction

Until 1980, urinary calculi passed spontaneously, were extracted by passage of a blind ureteric basket, observed, or were removed by open surgery.

Today, the options for the management of renal calculi are vastly different and numerous.

Notwithstanding the new treatment options, the indications for surgical intervention in renal stone disease have changed little.

These remain:

- Pain (ongoing)
- Obstruction
- Stone-associated infection
- Stones associated with decreased renal function
- Stones causing anuria
- Obstructive urosepsis
- Occupation (airline pilot, heavy machinery driver, traveller to remote regions, etc.)
- Others (transplant, organ donors)

The most common forms of renal stone surgery until 1980, open pyelolithotomy or nephrolithotomy, are now virtually extinct, being reserved for extremely complex calculi. The majority of "open stone" operations now are nephrectomy for burnt-out and complicated kidneys in the presence of stone, and most of these can be removed by laparoscopic nephrectomy.

Options for the Treatment of Renal Calculi

These include the following:

- Extracorporal shockwave lithotripsy (ESWL)
- Percutaneous nephrolithotomy (PCNL)
- Retrograde flexible ureterorenoscopic laser lithotripsy (FURS)
- Nephrolithotomy, ureterolithiotomy or nephrectomy
    - Open
    - Laparoscopic
    - Robot-assisted
- Oral dissolution
- Conservative management

Indications for PCNL

I find it easiest to define the stones most appropriately treated by PCNL as those that cannot be removed by ESWL, retrograde ureteroscopy, other forms of nephrolithotomy, or when these procedures have failed.

Historically, ESWL was described in 1980 by Chaussey and PCNL in 1981 by Alken and Wickham. Initially, ESWL was expensive and limited to specific sites in West Germany. It was not until 1984 that ESWL was performed outside Germany by Wickham et al.

As a result, PCNL, which required far less sophisticated and less expensive instrumentation, developed rapidly as the primary management for the majority of renal calculi, except for very large branched calculi, between 1981 and 1985.

When ESWL readily became available, it appeared that PCNL may become extinct.

However, it soon became clear that ESWL had its limitations. Experience demonstrated that the most appropriate calculi that could be safely treated by ESWL should be less than 2.5 cm in diameter, contained within a collecting system that drained freely and able to be completely fragmented by externally generated shockwaves. Cystine, brushite and calcium oxalate monohydrate calculi were refractory to ESWL. Generally, the higher the Hounsfield Unit (HU) of a calculus, the more refractory it is to ESWL. With PCNL, all calculi no matter what their HU measures are, can be fragmented by intracorporeal lithotripsy. Also, 30 % of patients retained residual stone fragments in the kidney following ESWL. This was obviously significant in relation to infection-related calculi and stone recurrence. Notwithstanding these indications and limitations, the majority of stones in developed countries were suitable for primary monotherapy by ESWL, as they were small and in normally draining collecting systems.

As PCNL removed calculi by a nephrocutaneous conduit, free distal drainage was not a prerequisite. Also, as all calculi, including those refractory to ESWL, could be broken by powerful lithotrites through a nephroscope, neither size nor composition presented a problem for PCNL. Anatomical access was the limiting factor.

PCNL became logical treatment for stones that were not suitable for ESWL or that had failed ESWL.

It was then a rational extension to combine the therapies so that a large stone obstructing a kidney could be debulked to leave an unobstructed system and the small peripheral fragments in difficult-to-access calyces could be cleared by subsequent ESWL.

Today, these smaller stones and fragments can be treated by ureteroscopy and laser FURS, as can calculi in obese patients in whom the distance from the skin to the kidney is too long for ESWL focus or the length of the nephroscope.

Current Indications for PCNL

- Staghorn calculi – large stone burden (>2.5 cm or 1.5 cm in the lower pole)
- Calculi contained within an obstructed collecting system (narrow PUJ, poorly draining lower pole calyces with narrow infundibulum, calculi within a horseshoe kidney)
- Infection-associated calculi, which require 100 % clearance to prevent recurrent infection
- Complex stones in urinary diversions (e.g. ileal conduit diversions) with large stone mass, infection and poor drainage
- Calculi refractory to ESWL, including cystine, brushite, calcium-oxalate and monohydrate calculi
- Calculi that require 100 % clearance for occupational regulations (airline pilots, military personnel, etc.)
- Congenital malformations with poor drainage (e.g. calyceal diverticulae, horseshoe kidney)
- Very large calculi impacted at or just below the pelviureteric junction and within the upper ureter, which are unsuitable for ureteroscopy
- Urinary obstruction requiring surgery to the collecting system (e.g. PUJ obstruction)

Contraindications to PCNL

- Unfit for general anaesthesia
- Untreated UTI
- Coagulation disorders
- Renal tumour
- Pregnancy
- Obesity
- Skeletal deformities (especially spinal)
- Ectopic or malrotated kidney
- Access prevented by surrounding organs, e.g. bowel/spleen

Schematic Comparison of ESWL and PCNL

ESWL

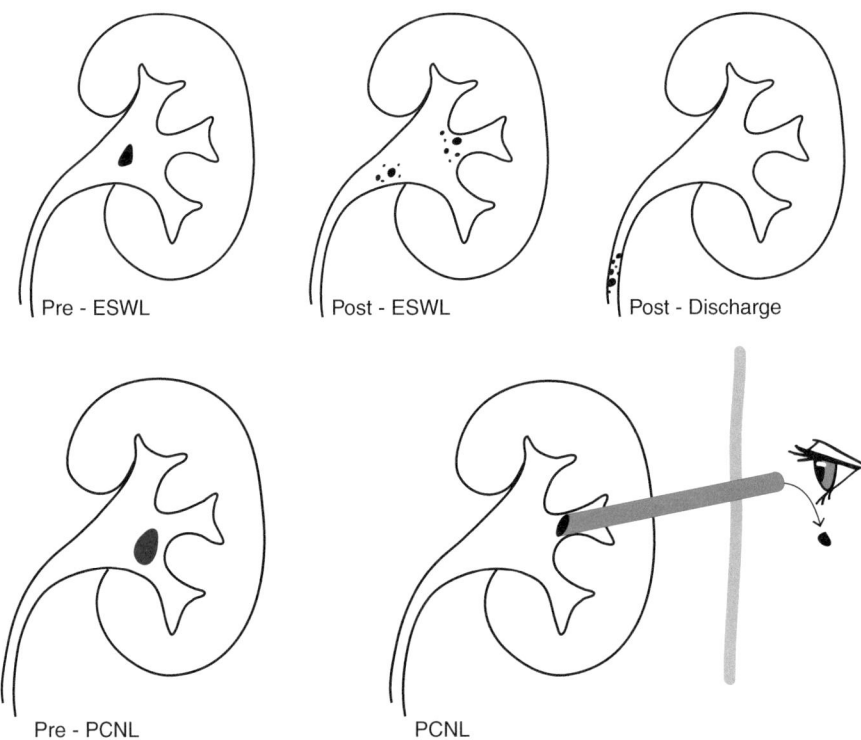

Fig 3.1 Schematic comparison of ESWL and PCNL

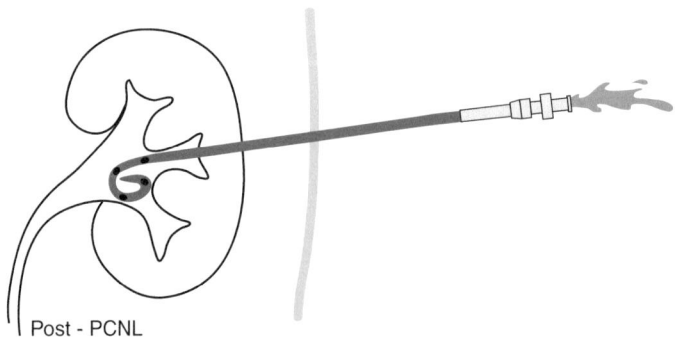

Fig 3.2 Free nephrostomy drainage following a PCNL

Preoperative Investigations Prior to PCNL

All patients require the following:

Laboratory

- Full blood examination
- Clotting profile
- Renal function tests
- Group and hold two units
- Midstream urine with culture and sensitivity

Radiological

- CT-KUB (and/or CT-IVP)
- Radioisotope renography, e.g. DMSA for kidney with thin or atrophic parenchyma

Patients requiring PCNL invariably have complex calculi or anatomy.

As continually emphasised in this manual, the most critical component of PCNL for both stone clearance and minimal morbidity is the creation of the nephrocutaneous access track.

There are two components to this track: the renal and the extra renal.

The ideal track is the shortest straightest track through the body wall, entering the thinnest and outermost portion of the kidney to access the collecting system through the tip of the calyx where the collecting system is best supported, parallel to the direction of that calyx, in the line of the intended surgery.

The best imaging modality to display the anatomy of the stone and the kidney is computed tomography (CT)

Conventional intravenous pyelography cannot accurately determine the position of a stone within a kidney, particularly as to whether it is positioned in an anterior or posterior calyx.

The minimal imaging investigation required prior to PCNL is a CT-KUB. This study outlines the body wall, the structures surrounding the kidney such as pleura bowel, liver or spleen and whether they lie in the path of the renal puncture. Within the kidney, the CT-KUB determines the size of the stone, the Hounsfield number which helps to predict stone density, and associated hydronephrosis, hydrocalycosis and parenchymal thickness. The CT-KUB gives a reasonable outline of the collecting system. However, if precise definition is required, a CT-IVP will outline the intrarenal anatomy and drainage.

Preoperative urinary tract ultrasound, in my experience, is of limited value.

It assesses large stones poorly, and does not show drainage or anatomy. Even with significant hydronephrosis in the presence of a large stone, an ultrasound image is unhelpful.

Urologists who are experienced with ultrasound find it most helpful intraoperatively for the renal puncture and stone location. Unfortunately, the majority of urologists do not have these ultrasound skills.

Summary: Preoperative Investigations for PCNL

- CT-IVU.
- CT KUB is sufficient if previous imaging studies such as intravenous urogram, retrograde pyelogram, nephrostogram or others are available, or the administration of contrast is medically contraindicated (i.e. renal failure allergy, etc.).
- Retrograde pyelogram – if no previous contrast study is available and the intravenous administration of contrast is contraindicated, the majority, if not all, information required for a safe PCNL can be attained from a CT-KUB. With antihistamine and steroid cover in consultation with the anaesthetist, a retrograde pyelogram can usually be performed if essential.
- Urine – microscopy, culture and sensitivity.
- FBE.
- Group and hold (cross match two units if anticipating multiple tracks).
- U and E, creatinine, eGFR.
- Clotting profile.

Consent

Consent should include a list of the complications of PCNL, including

1. Bleeding and possible transfusions (5–20 % depending on complexity)
2. Urosepsis (urine or blood 1–2 %)
3. Incomplete stone removal
4. Failed access
5. Cessation of PCNL prior to completion due to surgical complications (bleeding, lost track, perforation of collecting system or neighbouring organ such as pleura, lung, bowel, liver or spleen) with a view to a delayed secondary procedure
6. Radiological arterial embolisation (1–2 % – early postoperatively or delayed, e.g. arteriovenous fistula)
7. Further procedures, including ESWL, PCNL, FURS or rarely open nephrolithotomy or nephrectomy
8. Deep vein thrombosis (rare)

Preoperative Theatre Preparation

The urologist should have a working relationship with nursing and theatre technician staff, and notify them of specific requirements in advance.

Large Staghorn Calculus

- Inform theatre that it will be a long procedure
- Have both sonotrode and pneumatic lithoclast available
- Nephrostomies and other software required

Endoscopic Pyeloplasty

- Storz visual urethrotome
- Zero degree telescope lens
- Sickle "back cutting" cold knife
- Specify the size and make of double-J ureteric stent

Calyceal Diverticulum

- Ultrasonic lithotrite
- Target dilators
- "Mini Perc" instruments

Obese Patient, Horseshoe Kidney

- Multiple Amplatz sheaths to make "long sheath"
- Long nephroscope (rigid)
- Flexible cystoscope/nephroscope
- Holmium-YAG Laser
- Selection of ureteric baskets, e.g. Nitinol

Large Impacted Upper Ureteric Calculus

- Sonotrode
- Short rigid ureteroscope
- Multiple guide wires
- Flexible cystoscope/nephroscope
- Holmium-YAG Laser
- Mini-PCNL Set

Chapter 4
Percutaneous Nephrostomy

Percutaneous Nephrostomy (PCN)

Surgical Nephrostomy (SN)

Definition
A nephrostomy inserted by a surgeon or radiologist under general anaesthetic in the operating theatre at the time of PCNL to provide endoscopic access from the skin to the kidney, with the patient placed in the operative position.

Skinny Needle Surgical Nephrostomy (SNSN)

SNSN is of historical interest. It was routinely used by radiologists in the early days of PCN to introduce contrast into the renal pelvis to enable a targeted PCN. SNSN may be a useful fall back in cases such as a large upper ureteric calculus obstructing the kidney where it is not possible to bypass the stone or inject contrast into the kidney.

To perform SNSN, the patient lies prone. A long fine needle such as a lumbar puncture needle is inserted vertically through the skin in the lumbar triangle just lateral to the psoas directed to the predicted site of the renal pelvis. Once urine is aspirated, contrast is injected to outline the pelvic and calyceal anatomy. Then a routine PCN is inserted under screening.

Of course, in departments where ultrasound puncture is practised, this manoeuvre is redundant.

Radiological Nephrostomy (RN)

Definition
A nephrostomy inserted by a radiologist under local anaesthetic in the radiology department to establish percutaneous renal access for drainage, antegrade imaging, or antegrade manipulations such as the insertion of double J stents, basketing of calculi, balloon dilatations, etc.

Surgical Nephrostomy

In my experience, creating the nephrostomy access to the kidney is the most difficult aspect of PCNL for surgeons, particularly when learning PCNL.

PCN appears difficult.

Most manuals and individual surgeons have differing approaches and techniques for PCN.

Most urologists are more familiar with x-ray image intensifier (II) screening than ultrasound.

II is readily available in every hospital operating suite. This handbook describes surgical PCN using II screening.

Three-dimensional CT imaging for renal puncture is not readily available in most operating suites.

Puncture Technique

The PCN technique that works best for me is simple and requires only a basic C-arm II and biplanar fluoroscopy.

This technique of PCN is based on the location of an object in three-dimensional space using Cartesian coordinates.

In the Cartesian system, the "origin" is defined as the intersection of the X-, Y- and Z-axes. These axes represent the horizontal (Y), "straight ahead" (X) and vertical (Z) planes as they appear to the surgeon. The aim of this PCN technique is to create the Cartesian coordinates in the mind of the surgeon, where the "origin" is the anticipated entry point of the PCN needle into the kidney.

The spatial set up of the surgeon, kidney and image intensifier are critical for the understanding and employment of this technique.

By placing the surgeon, kidney and II monitor all on the same line, with the kidney between the surgeon and the monitor, the X (straight ahead) and Y (transverse) axes are automatically aligned.

Having established this set up with the X and Y axes, the surgeon needs only to calculate the angle and depth of the Z or vertical axis, to insert the needle into the calyx at the point of origin.

Fig. 4.1 The Cartesian spatial coordinates

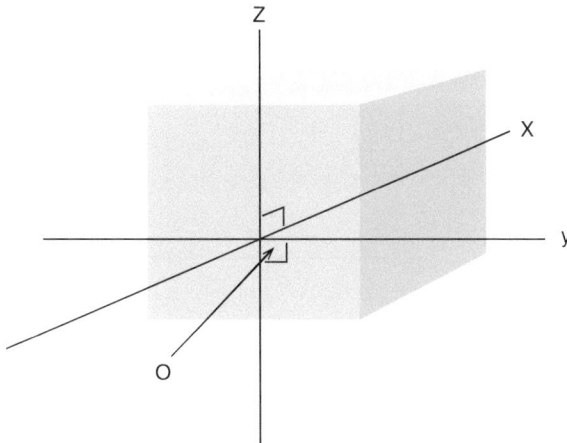

Fig. 4.2 Position of the surgeon, kidney and monitor to establish the X and Y axes for puncture

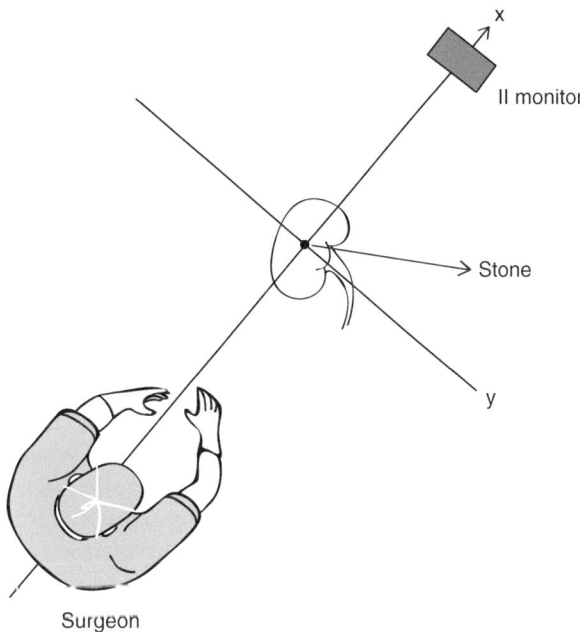

Having established the X and Y axes, the origin is vertically below the intersection of the X and Y axes on the skin. This point may be marked on the skin with the tip of a pair of artery forceps during II screening. By inserting the nephrostomy needle through the skin, parallel to the X-axis and at right angles to the Y-axis, the surgeon needs only to calculate the angle of the needle to the X-axis and the depth to which the needle will need to be advanced. With experience, this is usually simple and becomes almost second nature.

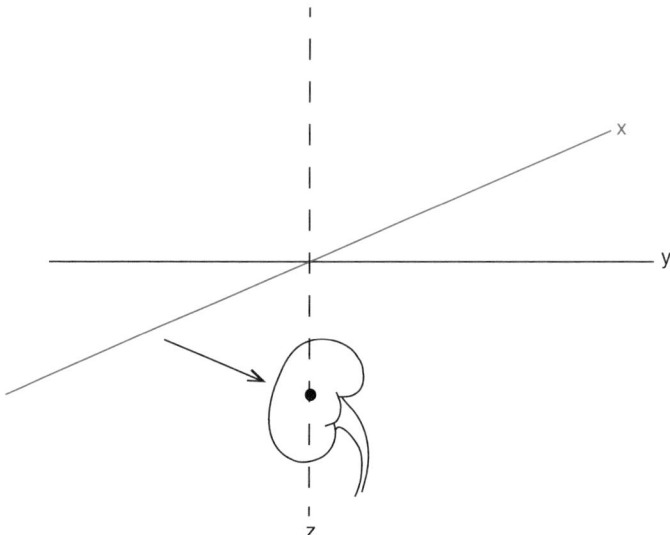

Fig. 4.3 The Z-axis, the depth and angle of which has to be estimated by the surgeon

Parallax

Parallax is a commonly used principle in astronomy, science and medicine. Parallax is defined as an apparent displacement of an object resulting from a change in the position from which it is viewed.

When applied to percutaneous renal puncture, the object that is "apparently displaced" is the needle tip, the "displacement" being relative to the kidney. The "observer" is the surgeon whose "eyes" are the fluoroscopy image from C-Arm camera as displayed on the x-ray monitors. As the surgeon rotates the C-Arm from the vertical position during fluoroscopy, with the axis of the beam focussed on the kidney, the needle will move relative to the kidney.

Parallax can be a difficult concept to understand and transfer to x-ray screening.

A simple model to illustrate parallax can be made by lining up three chairs in a straight line with a space between each chair. First, stand looking along the line of the chairs, each separated by a metre. This view represents the II screen from 12 o'clock, or vertical, when the needle tip is above or below, but not in the kidney.

Step 1

Imagine the middle chair to be the kidney and the other chairs the nephrostomy needle. This view mimics the II image from 12 o'clock. If this is viewed from 12 o'clock on the II, the "needle" appears to be in the kidney, whether it is superficial

Parallax 59

Fig. 4.4 Model for understanding parallax using three chairs

or deep to the kidney. Now take a few steps to the right. As you do focus your gaze on the middle chair, mimicking rotation of the C-Arm to 2 o'clock, with the x-ray beam focussed on the kidney. Return to the centre position and then move to the left ("10 o'clock"), observing that the relationships of the chairs reverse.

As you move, the chair closest to you (which represents a needle superficial to the kidney) appears to move away from you and the distant chair (the "deep needle") towards you. This is parallax. A gap appears to develop between the "kidney and needle", which widens, the further you walk around the chairs. Also, the chairs appear to rotate.

In both scenarios, the object that is furthest away from the observer (the deepest in the PCNL) is the one that appears to move the greater distance.

This model represents parallax when the needle is not in the kidney. If the needle is superficial to the kidney, the kidney is the object that will appear to "move" the furthest.

Parallax can also be utilised to confirm that the needle tip is in the kidney, or adjacent to the calculus. We call this absence of separation or relative movement "Reverse Parallax". When the observation point changes with rotation of the C-Arm, the objects will still appear to rotate, but they will not separate.

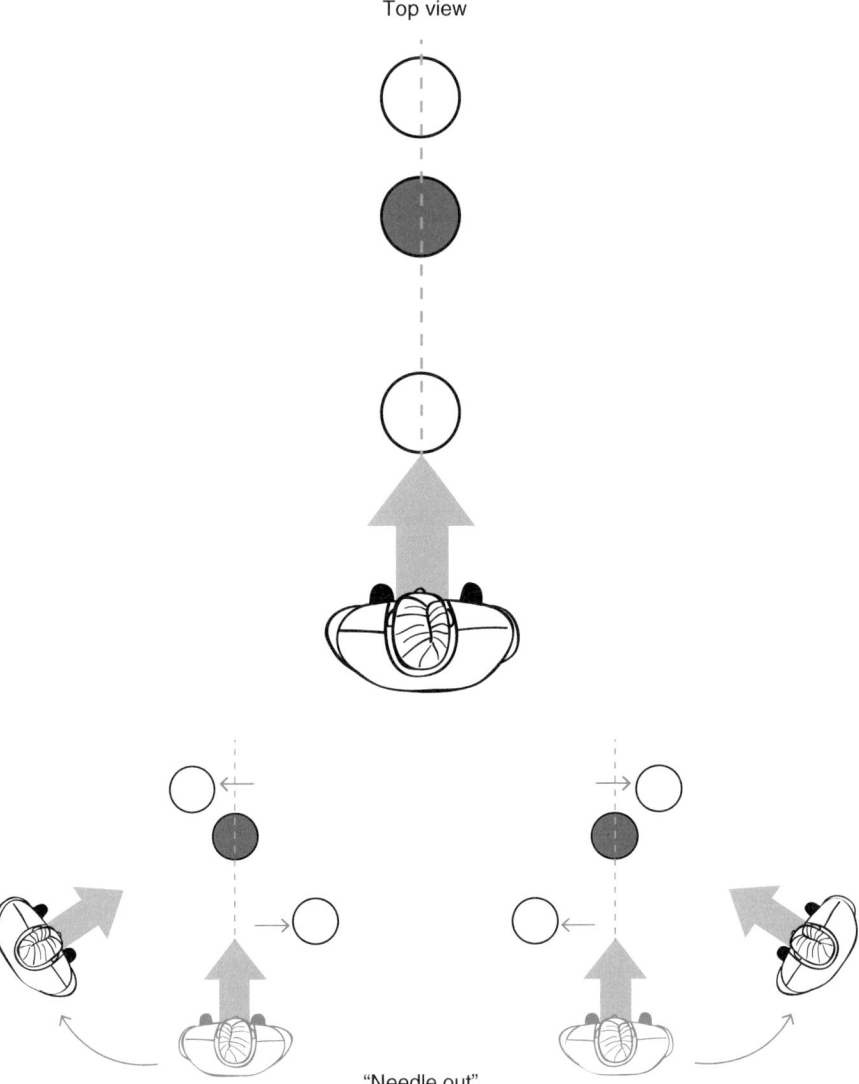

Fig. 4.5 Model for parallax when the needle is not in the calyx

Now place all the chairs in direct contact, with no spaces between and repeat the exercise. Although the three chairs will appear to rotate, no "gaps" will appear between them.

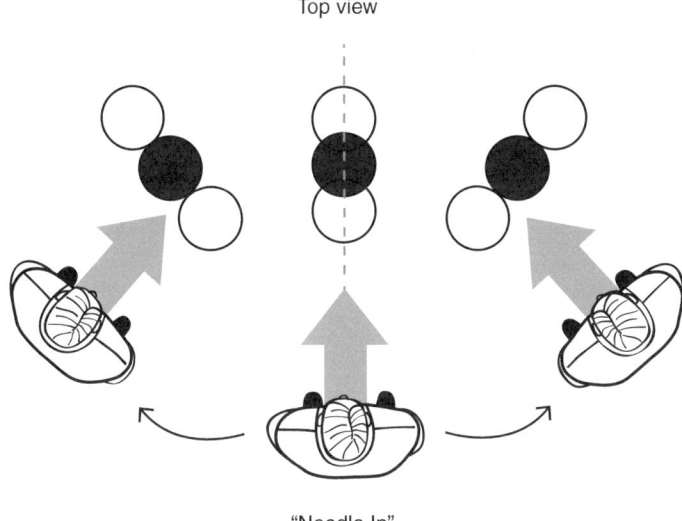

Fig. 4.6 "Reverse parallax model". No "gap" develops between the objects with a change of observer position, but they appear to rotate

So, when performing a nephrostomy, the surgeon inserts the puncture needle with the II camera vertical or at 12 o'clock. When it appears to be in the calyx on this A-P view, the radiographer will then, at the direction of the surgeon, slowly rotate the C-Arm on its axis, first to the right (2 o'clock) then back to the left of vertical (10 o'clock), continuously screening.

If the needle tip and the calyx move together with no gap developing between them, the needle is either in or just at the edge of the calyx. The surgeon can choose to further advance the needle or remove the stylet.

If a gap appears, the needle is not in the calyx.

If, as the gap widens on rotation of the C-Arm, the needle appears to move further than the kidney then the needle is deep to the kidney.

The surgeon then removes the needle and repunctures along a more superficial track, with the II camera at 12 o'clock.

Similarly, if the needle appears to move less, it is superficial to the kidney, so the needle is reinserted more vertically and deeply.

In practice, the application and understanding of parallax requires experience.

"Reverse parallax" is an easy concept and very helpful to confirm that the needle is correctly in the kidney. Utilising parallax when the needle is not in the kidney is a more difficult concept to grasp, but becomes easy with practise. I suggest you discuss parallax with your radiologist. Radiologists are very familiar with the concept of parallax and teaching the skill, which is how I learned it.

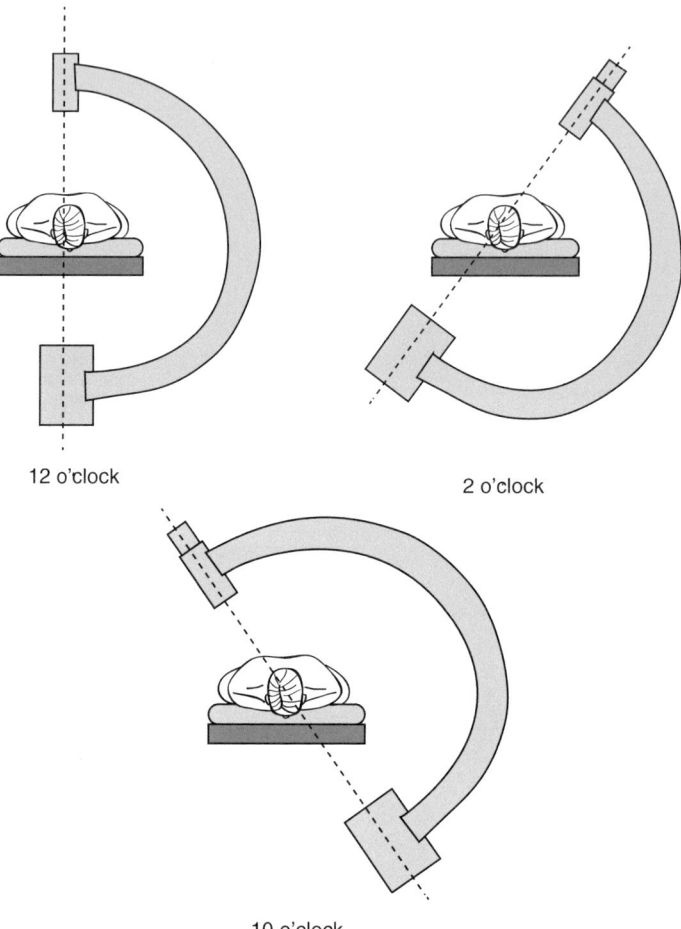

Fig. 4.7 Parallax in practise, the C-Arm "looking at" or "viewing" the kidney from 10, 12 and 2 o'clock

I have found that the insertion of the needle along the vertical vector is easily learnt by experience. Only occasionally do I find it necessary to rotate the C-Arm (parallax) to judge the depth and angle of needle insertion in a patient of average build.

Needle puncture in thin and obese patients can be challenging. In both, estimating depth can be deceptive. I find I overestimate the depth in thin patients and underestimate the depth in a large patient, so my initial puncture is often too deep in thin patients and too superficial in an obese case.

Fig. 4.8 Nephrostomy needle superficial to the kidney in an obese patient. The needle appears to be in the calyx on the 12 o'clock (vertical) image on the II. This first puncture is represented by the pale, shaded needle. After establishing that the needle tip is superficial by parallax, the needle (the dark needle) is reinserted more vertically and deeply

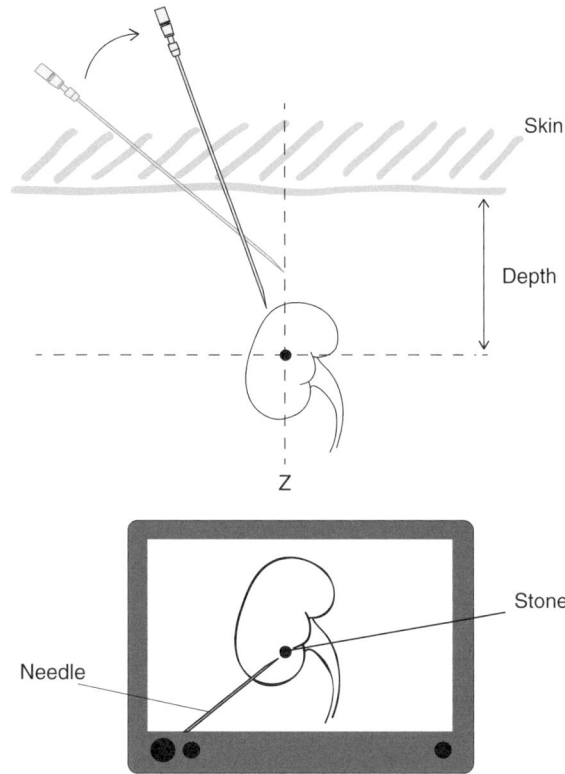

For example, when performing PCNL on an obese patient, it is very easy to place the needle superficial to the kidney. The AP image on the II monitor does not show depth. Deep kidney: e.g., obese patient, horseshoe or malrotated kidney, skeletal abnormality.

Conversely, in a very thin or a paediatric patient, the initial puncture is often deep into the kidney.

These variations in anatomy and depth need to be borne in mind by the surgeon and anticipated prior to PCN. They become apparent with practice. They should be utilised in conjunction with other features that assist the surgeon in knowing when the needle is in the kidney, such as needle movement with respiration, the "half moon" sign and parallax.

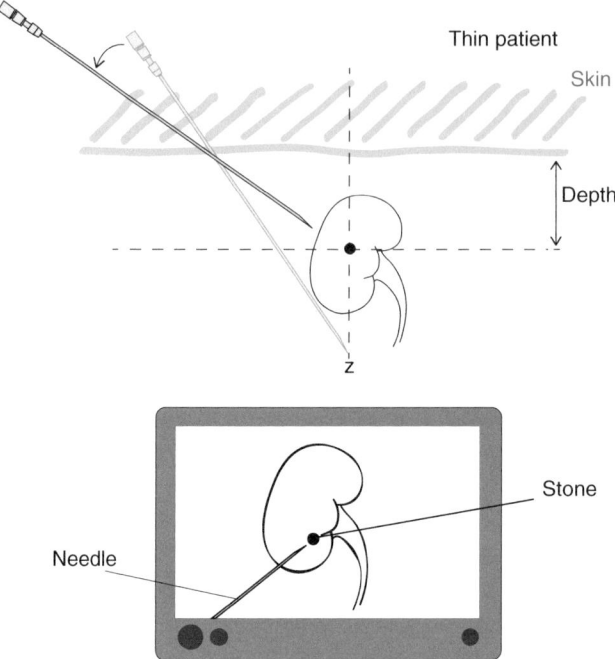

Fig. 4.9 Nephrostomy needle deep into the kidney in a thin patient. On the 12 o'clock view, it appears to be in the kidney. The pale needle of the first puncture attempt is confirmed as deep into the kidney using parallax. The needle is removed and reinserted (dark needle) on a more shallow and less angled trajectory.

Technique of Percutaneous Renal Puncture

I use a standard technique of cystoscopy and ureteric catheterisation with the patient positioned in lithotomy, followed by the renal puncture with the patient placed prone on the operating table. The prone position provides access to a wider area of renal surface and shorter track than the supine position. As almost all of my PCNLs are for complex staghorn calculi and usually require multiple tracks, I do not use the supine approach. However, I do not have a negative attitude towards supine PCNL. Prone works best for me and the calculi I manage.

Lithotomy Position

Step 2

1. Panendoscopy
2. Retrograde catheter (Six French open-ended catheter with proximal Leur lock) passed under II screening so that the tip is well into the renal pelvis or upper

Fig. 4.10 Method of fixation of the ureteric catheter before turning the patient prone

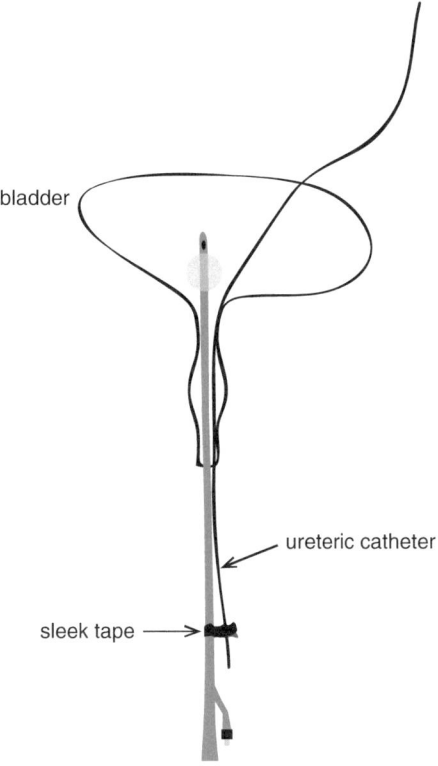

calyx. NB: when the patient is transferred from lithotomy to the prone position, it is common for the distal tip of the catheter to migrate proximally towards the bladder for 2–3 cms, hence the necessity for the catheter tip to be placed well within the renal pelvis or upper pole calyx at the time of insertion. If the catheter tip migrates into the upper ureter, contrast distension and opacification can be compromised.

3. 16 French two-way Foley urethral catheter
4. RGC taped securely to the foley catheter using waterproof adhesive (SLEEK), creating a "mesentery" between the two catheters.
5. An empty 20 ml syringe is inserted into Leur lock and taped to the urethral catheter as well. This maintains sterility of the Leur lock lumen and prevents inadvertent movement of the RGC during patient transfer.
6. Contrast must not be injected while the patient is in lithotomy if the operation is for stone. Exceptions are endoscopic endopyelotomy, where there is confusion or doubt as to whether the catheter is within the kidney, difficulty in passing a guide wire, suspicion of ureteric trauma or obstruction or ureteric anatomical variations such as bifid ureters.

Prone Position of the Patient

Patient Safety

Both surgeon and anaesthetist must be familiar with the risks of surgery in the prone position.

(a) Facial sponge and support:
   A facial sponge box or similar support should be used to support the patient's head, neck and endotracheal tube and avoid pressure to the face.
(b) Padding of pelvis, chest and ankles:
   The patient should lie with pillows separating the chest and pelvis from the operating table.
(c) Patient positioning for optimal access:
   I prefer the "free style swimmer" position for optimal access from the flank to the kidney.

In this position, the arm on the ipsilateral or stone side is elevated forward and the contralateral arm is along the side of the patient's torso. This rotates the shoulders, and hence the chest, opening the infracostal angle. As the ipsilateral arm is also the most accessible to the anaesthetist, it should be the site for vascular lines.

The body is placed gently concave away from the stone and the pelvis tilted downwards by placing both legs towards the contralateral side of the table.

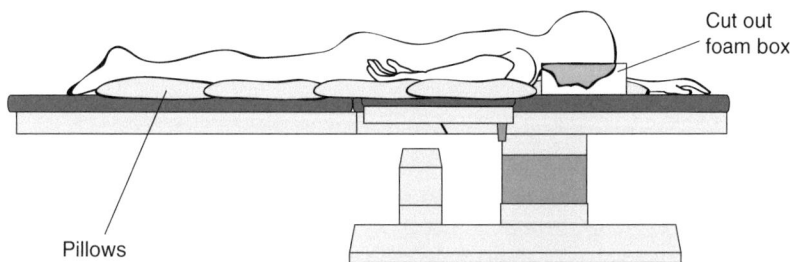

Fig. 4.11 Patient position with urinary tract clear of table pylon to facilitate II screening with pillows supporting the chest, hips and ankles and the head and endotracheal tube in a cut out foam box

With this arrangement, the legs angulate the pelvis, further opening up the space between the chest and the pelvic bones, facilitating infracostal access.

I place a triangular sponge under the kidney, slightly angulating the torso upwards from the table, to present the posterior calyces more end on.

Occasionally, this kidney bolster can displace the kidney cephalad, in which case it can be removed and done without.

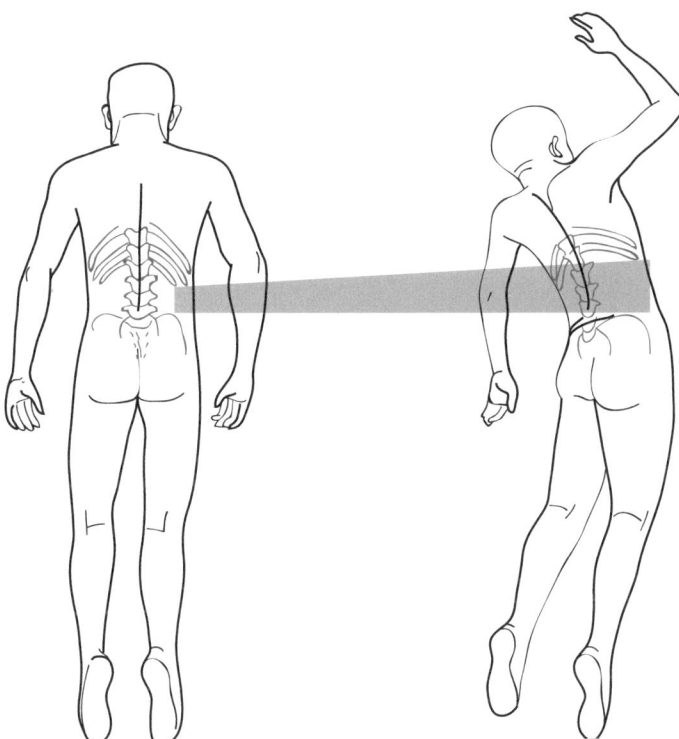

Fig. 4.12 "Free Style Swimmer" position to obtain maximum needle access from the flank. Note how the angulations open up the space between the pelvis and the ribs.

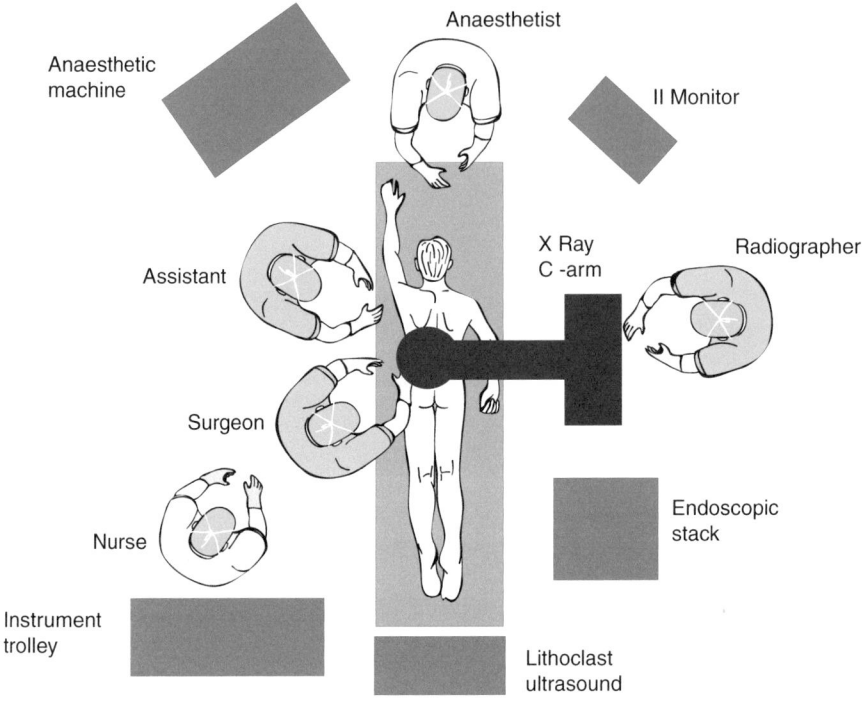

Fig. 4.13 Theatre set-up for PCNL

Theatre Set-Up

(a) Positioning of personnel and equipment

The most critical factor when using the Cartesian puncture technique is for the surgeon, the point of access into the kidney and the II monitor to be in a direct line.

This enables the surgeon to stand so that when looking ahead across the patient to the monitor, he is looking along the *X*-axis of the Cartesian coordinates. The *Y*-axis is naturally perpendicular to *X*, leaving only the depth or *Z*-axis to calculate.

(b) Patient and equipment set-up

The anaesthetic staff and their equipment are at the head of the patient and to the surgeon's side. This allows for the II monitor to be in the direct view of the surgeon, over and behind the patients' shoulder.

The surgeon stands on the operative side of the patient. The II monitor, II, C-Arm and endoscopic "stack" (camera monitor, light source) are on the opposite side of the patient.

Stone fragmentation equipment (ultrasonic and ballistic) is placed at the foot of the patient.

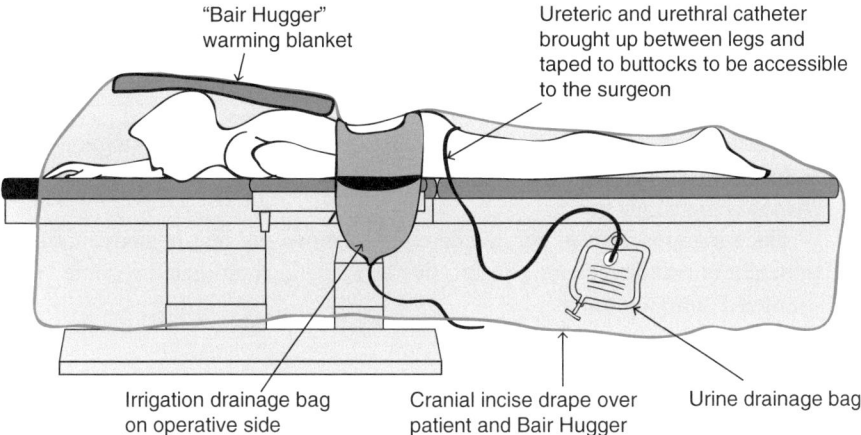

Fig. 4.14 Draping for PCNL in the prone position

(c) Patient draping:
It is critical that the patient remains dry and warm throughout the PCNL.

Temperature loss from convection and cooling from irrigant and wet drapes is significant and can be rapid. Whenever possible, patients should be warmed with a "Bair Hugger" warming device. This can be taped onto the patients back above the 10th rib posteriorly.

I prefer to use a craniofacial drape for PCNL as it is waterproof, easily applied and has a transparent adhesive window that attaches to the skin over the puncture site. Before applying the drape, the urethral catheter and the attached ureteric catheter hub are brought dorsally between the legs so that the ureteric catheter can be taped to the patient's buttock on the operative side. The ureteric catheter is then brought through a small incision in the craniofacial drape after the drapes are applied. This gives the surgeon direct ureteric access for the passage of guide wires and the injection of contrast or methylene blue infusions.

After securing the ureteric catheter to the buttock, the craniofacial drape is attached with the irrigant-collecting bag on the surgeon side. The dependant tip of this bag is drained into a bucket via attached tubing.

A small hole is made with scissors in the craniofacial drape over the buttock where the ureteric catheter can be felt and the ureteric catheter hub is brought through the drape into the operative site. Minimum volume extension tubing is attached to the Leur lock on the RGC, for contrast infusion.

Prior to the PCN puncture, it is essential for the surgeon to check all the PCNL equipment, in particular the nephroscope. The urologist must also confirm that the ultrasonic lithotrite, irrigant pump and the pneumatic lithotrite are all functioning. If they are not, they must be fixed before commencing the puncture.

There is no time after the puncture has commenced to repair malfunctioning endoscopes or lithotrites.

All saline infusions must be warmed.

(d) Percutaneous renal puncture:

To me the most critical step of the percutaneous puncture is the surgeon positioning himself such that the point of entry to the kidney and II are on the same X-axis as the surgeon.

Once positioned, it is my practice, not to move my feet or body, until the puncture is completed. As a result, the X, Y and Z coordinates become "programmed" into my mind.

Step One:
Surgeon, patient, stone and II are "lined up" on the X-axis.

Step Two:
II C-Arm is placed vertically above the kidney and the stone located. A "snap shot" image is taken and stored for future reference before contrast is injected.

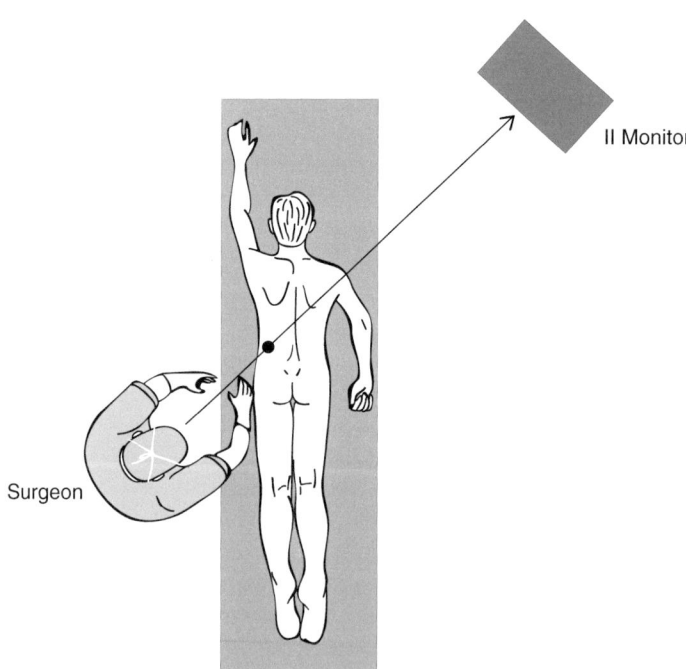

Fig. 4.15 Surgeon setting up the X and Y axes of the Cartesian coordinates by having the stone along the line of sight to the II monitor

Technique of Percutaneous Renal Puncture

Step Three:
Contrast (a mixture of saline, contrast and methylene blue) is slowly infused by the surgeon or assistant under continuous II screening.

While screening, the surgeon holds a scalpel with a fine pointed blade so that the axis of the scalpel handle and blade are parallel to the X-axis, and the direction of the calyx to be entered.

The blade is placed, under II screening, over and parallel to the calyx. Then, also under II screening, the blade is slowly withdrawn towards the surgeon. A 2–3 mm skin puncture is made by the scalpel tip approximately 5 cm towards the surgeon from the vertical point where the stone is located on II.

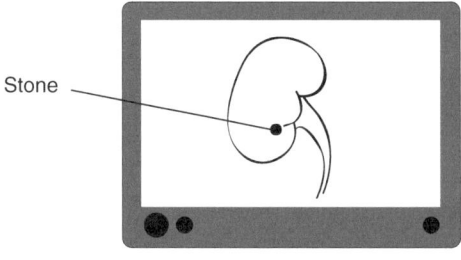

Fig. 4.16 Stored pre-contrast image of calculus

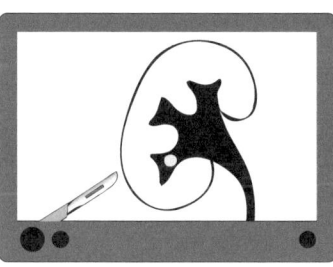

Fig. 4.17 II screening during injection of contrast via RGC

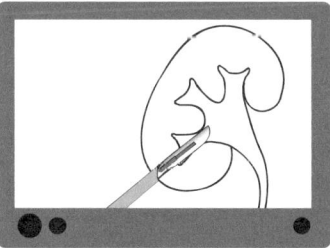

Fig. 4.18 Using the scalpel blade and handle to plan the direction of the nephrostomy puncture

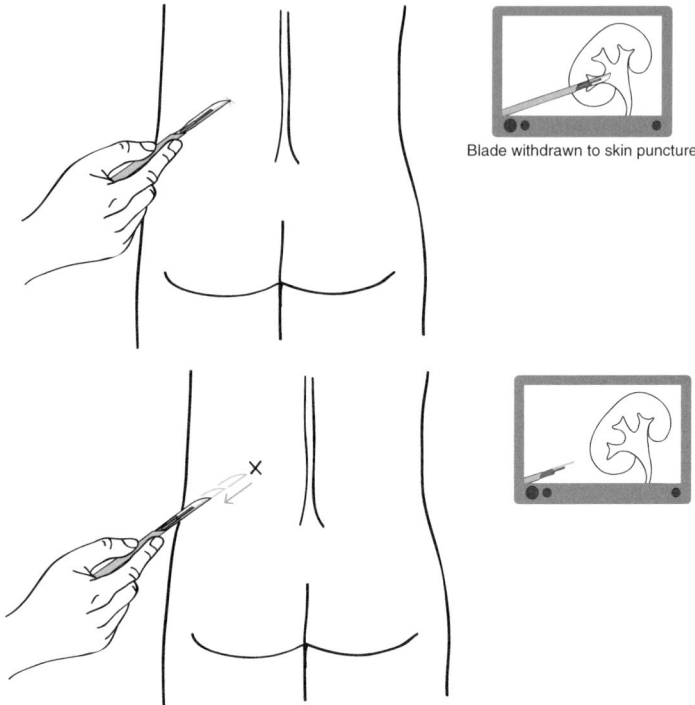

Fig. 4.19 Withdrawal of the scalpel blade during II screening to plan puncture direction. When the tip of the scalpel is at the selected skin entry point, a small 2–3 mm full thickness skin puncture is made in the anticipated direction and angle for the needle puncture

It is important that the scalpel is withdrawn along the line of the calyx or intended puncture.

Be aware, it is easy and may be very confusing if the II image is on the monitor "flipped" or transposed. If this is unrecognised, it is nearly impossible to puncture the kidney.

Be sure the Calyx is pointing towards you and that the scalpel moves in the same direction on the monitor as it does in your hand.

The calyx to be entered should be identified prior to surgery on the preoperative CT scans.

When puncturing for a single stone or calculus in a calyceal diverticulum, one is attempting to enter that calyx directly. In the case of a more complex stone such as a staghorn calculus, the primary puncture should be the route that will give maximum clearance of the stone bulk through one track, even if not complete clearance. If the puncture is for other pathology such as endopyelotomy or a large upper ureteric stone, then the calyx selected should be the one that leads directly the area requiring surgery, e.g. PUJ. These cases usually require mid zone or upper pole punctures.

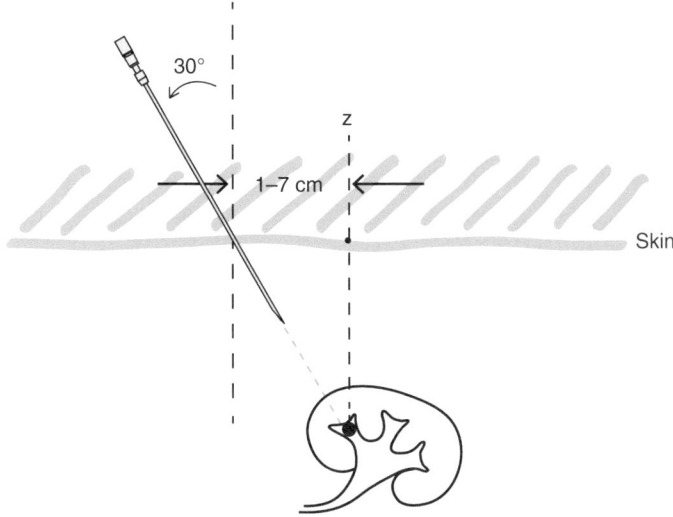

Fig. 4.20 The initial needle puncture, usually 30° off the vertical plane, through the skin "stab"

(e) Puncture and insertion of needle:
The needle should be placed over the kidney, under II screening, parallel to the calyx and over the stone. It is then withdrawn, approximately 5 cm, as was the scalpel blade when making the first skin puncture. It is important that the surgeon does not move, thereby retaining the "pre-programmed" spatial coordinates of the puncture.

When making the skin incision, the scalpel handle and blade should be inserted at the same angle as the needle.

A small skin incision of 2–3 mm should be made parallel to Langer's lines. The needle and sheath are introduced through the skin for approximately 1 cm. The needle is then "wiggled" from side to side, to ensure that there is no rib in the needle path, or tough dermis that might damage the outer needle sheath.

The surgeon should then ask the anaesthetist to stop respiration in inspiration, to maximally displace the kidney downwards. The needle hub is held between the index finger and the forefinger, with the thumb over the proximal Leur lock.

The needle is advanced at 30° from the vertical, parallel to the "straight head" X-axis, guided by the image on the monitor. As most posterior calyces face 30° posteriorly, the needle will tend to enter parallel to a posterior calyx. Under continuous II screening, the surgeon should advance the needle towards the tip of the calyx. With experience, one will often "feel" the tip of the needle as it penetrates the capsule of the kidney, and may also observe a calyceal spasm. This indicates that the tip of the needle is just at the edge of the collecting system. The spasm produces the "half-moon sign" as the calyceal neck reflexly contracts. At this point, advance the needle another 2–3 mm to enter the calyx. You may feel a small "give" as the needle enters the lumen of the calyx.

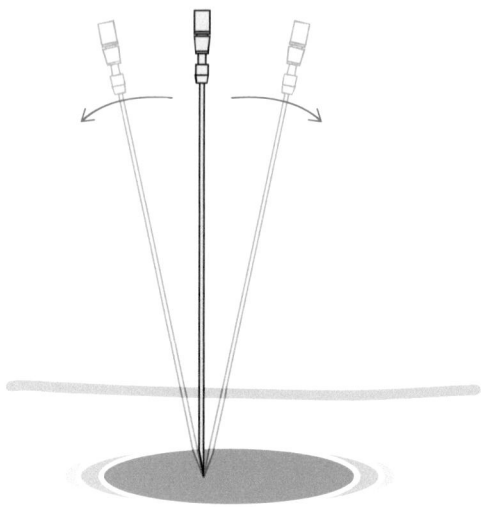

Fig. 4.21 When the needle is in the kidney, it will move externally with respiration

Now release your grasp on the needle and ask the anaesthetist to resume respiration.

If the needle is within the kidney, it will move with respiration. If not, the hub will not move.

This sign confirms that the needle is in the kidney, but not necessarily within the collecting system.

(f) Final needle placement:

If the surgeon feels that the needle tip is within the calyx, (having felt the "give" sign), it should not be advanced further. Otherwise, if over advanced, the needle tip may puncture and exit the opposite side of the calyx.

At this stage, the stylet and needle should be withdrawn from the teflon needle sheath.

If contrast and methylene blue freely exit from the needle sheath, a hydrophilic 0.38 "straight ahead" floppy tip guide wire is inserted under II guidance and threaded down the ureter if possible.

If not, then as much guide wire as possible should be coiled in the kidney to give stability for subsequent dilatation. Floppy hydrophilic guide wires will readily coil in the pelvis and around a calculus.

If the surgeon is not confident that the needle is in the collecting system, and there has not been a calyceal spasm or "pop" or "give", and yet the needle appears to be in on II and parallax screening, advance the needle a further half a centimetre, as the tip may have been just short of the collecting system.

At this stage, the stylet and needle should be removed from the sheath.

Technique of Percutaneous Renal Puncture

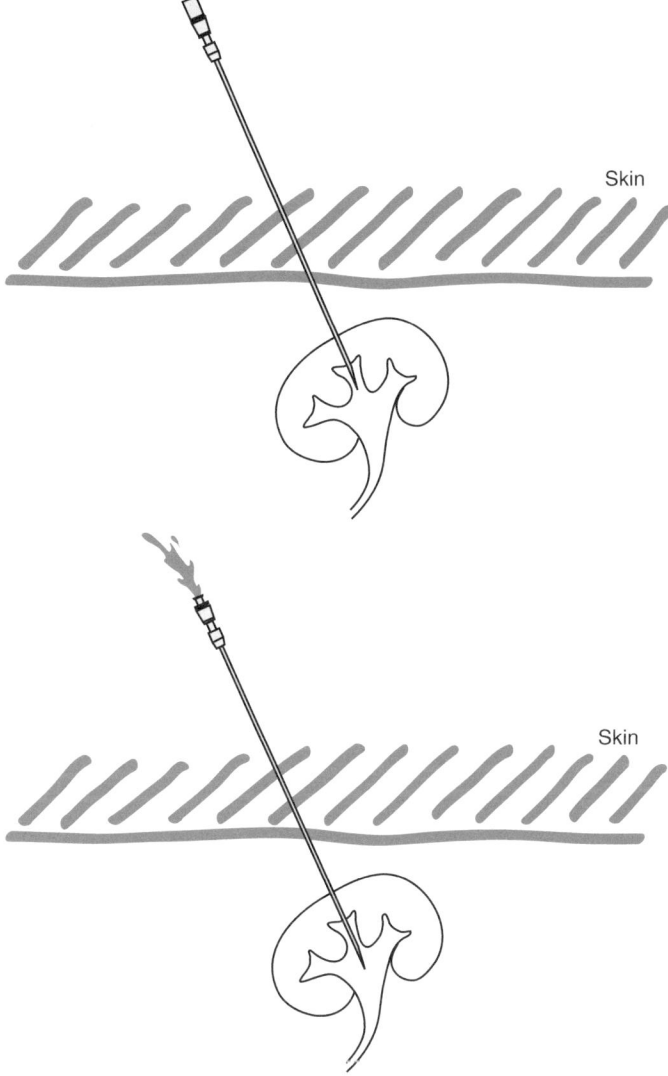

Fig. 4.22 Methylene blue coloured contrast flowing from the needle sheath after removal of the needle, confirming successful entry into the collecting system

If the stylet is removed but no contrast flows from the sheath, under NO circumstances should the needle be reintroduced into the sheath. With respiration, the sheath will kink. Reinsertion of the needle will invariably pierce and may transect the sheath.

Fig. 4.23 Guide wire introduced through the sheath under II screening

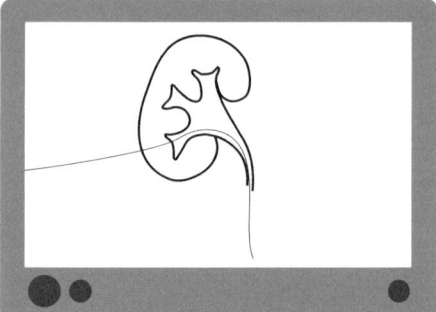

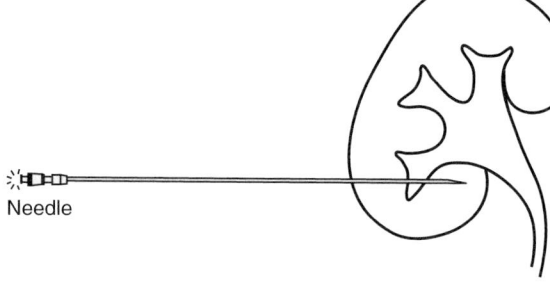

Fig. 4.24 "Through and through" puncture by the nephrostomy needle, the needle tip has traversed the calyx and punctured and exited into or through the parenchyma

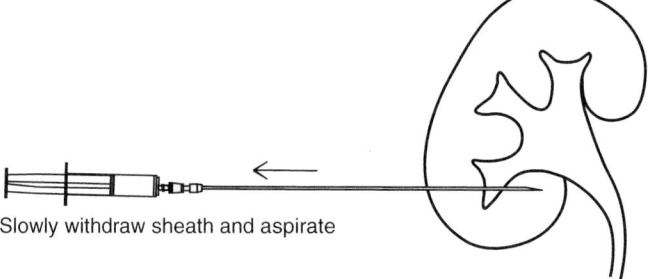

Fig. 4.25 Aspiration to assess whether the needle had passed through the calyx

It is often the case that the needle, which appears to be in the collecting system on the AP view, has traversed the calyx and pierced the contralateral side of the calyx and possibly through into the retroperitoneum.

The surgeon should attach a small 20 cc syringe to the Leur lock at the proximal end of the needle sheath and aspirate very gently, withdrawing the needle sheath at the same time.

If the tip of the sheath enters the lumen of the calyx, it will "flash" blue contrast.

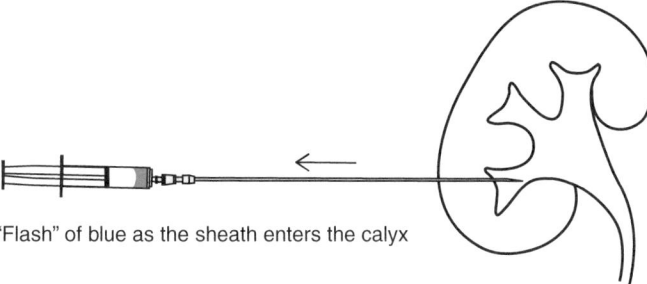

Fig. 4.26 Positive "flash" sign as the tip of the needle sheath is slowly drawn into the lumen of the calyx

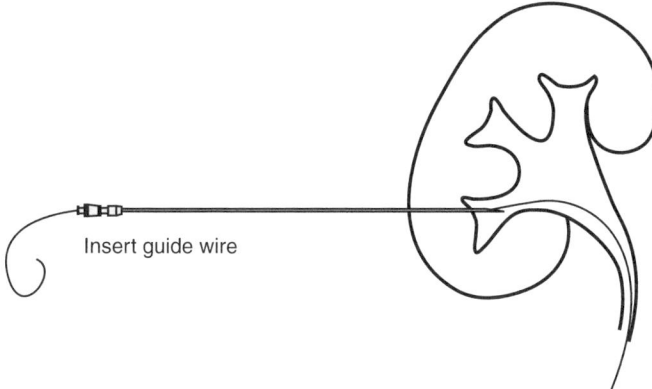

Fig. 4.27 Insertion of guide wire under II screening following positive "flash" test

When a "flash" occurs, the syringe is removed and a guide wire inserted into the collecting system. It is very important to withdraw slowly and cease immediately when methylene blue is seen. The calyceal lumen may only be a few millimetres wide, making it very easy to extract the sheath from the proximal wall of the lumen.

Occasionally, when only a small volume is aspirated, and is bloody, it is not possible to be sure whether it is pure blood or blood stained urine. In this scenario, I ask the radiographer to take a "snapshot". If the aspirate is urine, it will be radioopaque, so the contrast filled needle sheath will show on the II. We call this the "Thread Sign". If the sheath is not opacified, it is still worth gently inserting a floppy-tipped guide wire as it will occasionally still go into the collecting system. If both these manoeuvres fail, the sheath must be removed and the kidney re-punctured.

Failure to aspirate contrast suggests that the needle has punctured the kidney lateral or deep to but not through the calyx, or is outside the kidney. The latter is often seen when the kidney is very deep.

When no contrast can be aspirated on withdrawal, the needle and sheath should be withdrawn completely and a new puncture performed.

Assuming the surgeon has not moved (retaining the "3D coordinates"), it is a simple procedure to reinsert the needle with the outer end of the needle angled slightly further from the vertical, so the tip of the needle enters the kidney more superficially than the previous puncture. From experience, the majority of failed punctures that "look-in" on the II but are not, have passed deep to the calyx.

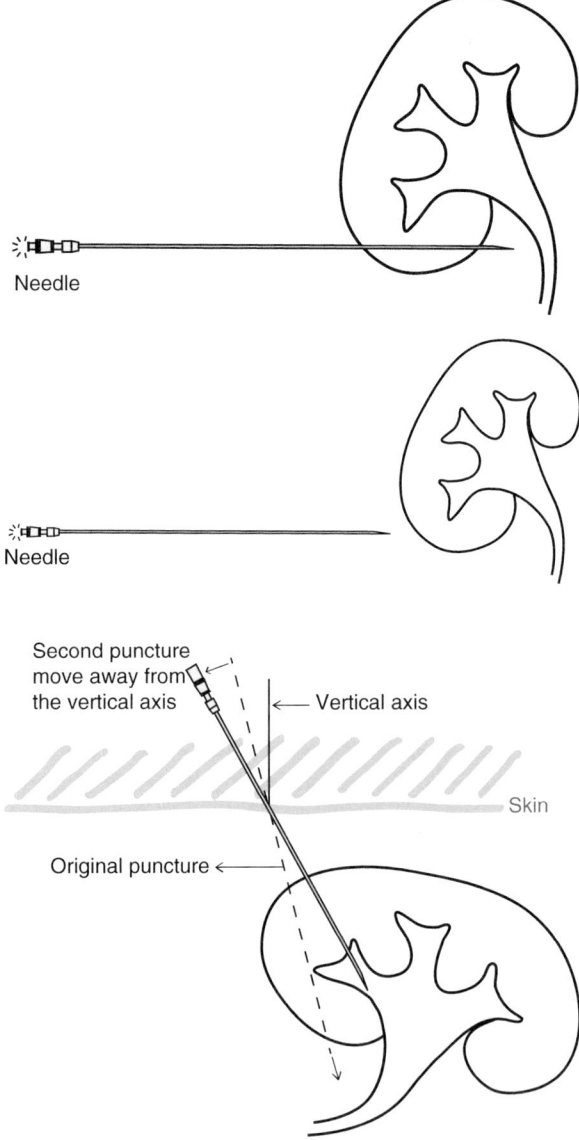

Fig. 4.28 Negative "flash" test – no contrast aspirated during withdrawal of the needle, where the needle has not punctured the collecting system

Fig. 4.29 Re-puncture at a different angle depending on parallax screening; in this case, a more superficial angle

Technique of Percutaneous Renal Puncture

The change of angulation usually results in the needle entering the calyx.

If in doubt, "parallax" can be employed.

Using parallax, one will then be able to decide whether the needle tip is superficial or deep to the calyx.

There are two objects of interest: the tip of the needle and the calyx (or targeted stone). Whichever is deepest will move farthest during "parallax" screening. With this knowledge, the surgeon adjusts the angle and depth of the needle path accordingly.

(g) "Through and through" calyceal puncture:

When the nephrostomy needle has punctured the calyx, and also inadvertently gone too deep and continued through the kidney, slow retraction of the sheath and aspiration of the methylene blue ("flash sign") will confirm that the tip of the sheath is in the collecting system. However, when advancing a straight hydrophilic guide wire, in spite of the sheath tip definitely being within the collecting system, the tip of the guide wire may persist in continuing through the original puncture track out of the kidney instead of along the lumen of the calyx.

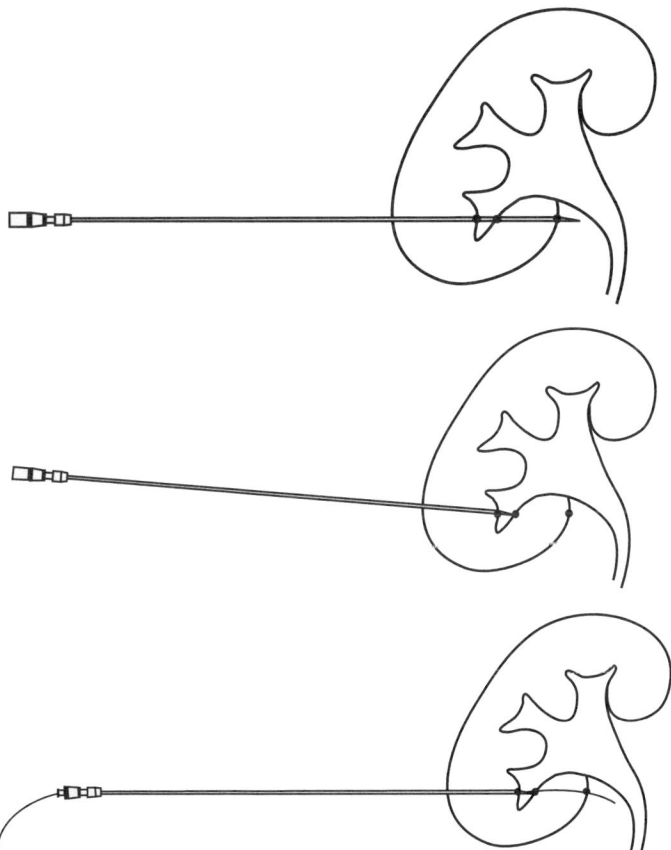

Fig. 4.30 In spite of a positive "flash" test, the guide wire exits through the puncture hole rather than advancing along the lumen of the calyx

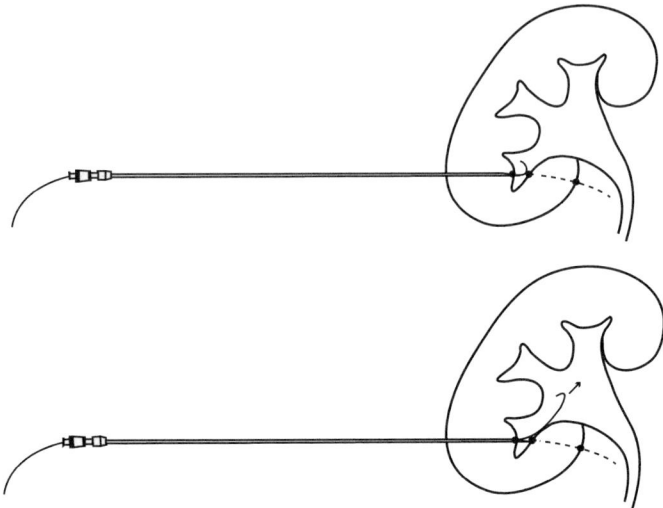

Fig. 4.31 The straight wire is replaced by a J wire that coils, preventing it exiting from the deep puncture track

This is frustrating and usually obvious by the II image of the guide wire, which coils outside the kidney in the retroperitoneum.

To avoid the wire exiting the kidney, remove the hydrophilic guide wire and insert a "J" wire. The "J" wire tip curls immediately as it leaves the end of the nephrostomy needle sheath.

As a result of this coiling, the tip is not directed straight ahead, so the wire cannot exit the puncture and the coil advances through the calyx and infundibulum.

Once the J wire is confirmed to be within the infundibulum or renal pelvis on II, the needle sheath can be advanced over the J wire so that the sheath is now safely within and parallel to the collecting system and away from the "through and through" puncture.

If following a puncture, the needle is removed and no contrast can be aspirated, under NO circumstance should contrast be injected through the sheath. In this situation, the needle sheath will not be in the kidney. Injected contrast will extravasate around the kidney in the perinephric space, obliterating the radiological anatomy, preventing further punctures. If only a small amount has extravasated, it may resorb in 5–10 min or can sometimes be diluted sufficiently to re-image the calyx by injecting normal saline through the sheath.

Generally though, perirenal contrast cannot be flushed away, resulting in termination of the procedure.

If bubbles extrude in or around a puncture, they usually signify trouble! Almost always one has punctured the pleura or bowel. Be wary of bubbles!

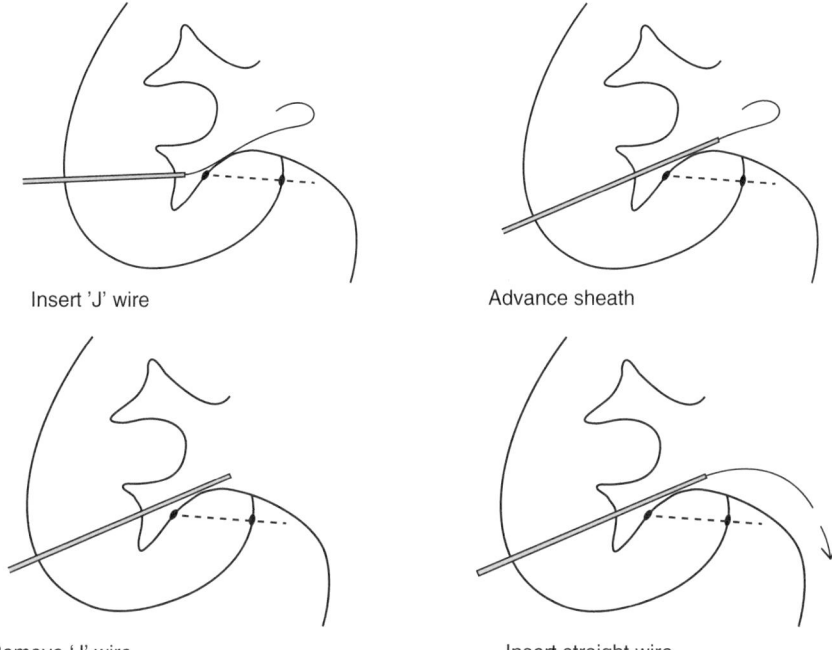

Fig. 4.32 Guide wire exchange sequence to replace the J wire with a straight wire after gaining stable access to the collecting system

Radiological Nephrostomy

Definition

A radiological nephrostomy (RN) is a percutaneous nephrostomy inserted in the X-ray department under local anaesthetic.

The commonest indications are urosepsis, malignant anuria, antegrade insertion of stent, drainage of pyonephrosis or pyocalyx, relief of ureteric colic, post ESWL for the relief of obstruction secondary to a "stein strasse", or electively prior to PCNL. In the latter, the RN will provide drainage of urosepsis and may become the conduit for contrast infusion at the time of PCNL.

As a RN is performed with the patient awake and usually sitting up, (in other words, not in the prone PCNL or operative position) and often without distention of the calyces by retrograde catheter injection, a RN is rarely optimal for use as an access track for a complex PCNL.

The track of a RN tends to be long and angulated and often enters the collecting system medially through an infundibulum or the renal pelvis. This is not a criticism of RN, it is a clinical reality.

Therefore, even in the presence of a RN, I manage the patient as if the RN were absent. In other words, the patient should still have a cystoscopy, retrograde catheter and then a PCNL performed in theatre as a single-stage procedure. The RN should remain in situ until the new track is created.

The exceptions to this "rule" include cases such as urinary diversions, where there is no retrograde access, or anatomical deformities, particularly in cases of neurogenic bladder and spina bifida, where the only method of instilling contrast is through a RN. I have the RN inserted at least 48 h prior to the PCNL. These patients usually have complex obstructed infection stones. The early nephrostomy not only guarantees access, but decompresses unsuspected obstructive urosepsis, making the definitive PCNL safer with respect to infection and septic shock.

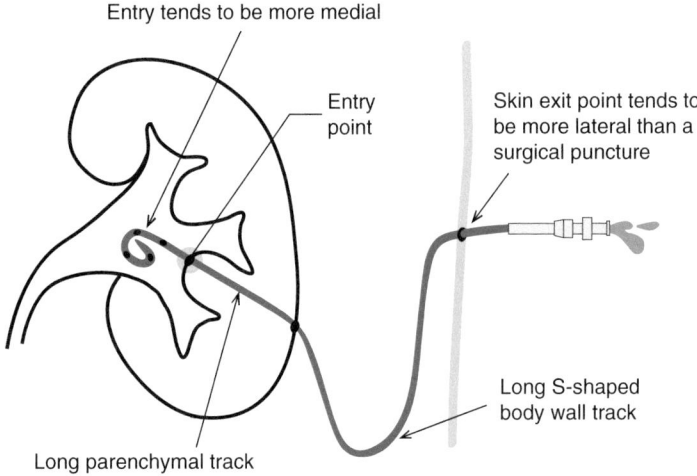

Fig. 4.33 Radiological nephrostomy

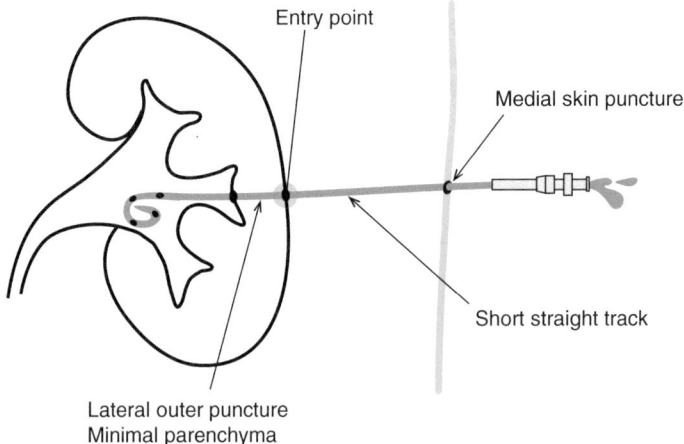

Fig. 4.34 Surgical nephrostomy

Chapter 5
Routine PCNL

Most urologists have their own techniques for track dilatation, stone fragmentation and removal.

This chapter describes my technique of establishing a track for PCNL.

In spite of variations in instrumentation and techniques, the principles of PCNL and track creation remain constant.

The overriding requirement for successful PCNL is unhurried patience and avoidance of force.

Ignoring these principles invariably results in complications or early termination of the procedure.

This chapter describes patient positioning, percutaneous puncture of the kidney and the introduction of a stable guide wire.

I have two aims when placing a guide wire.

- Firstly, that the guide wire is passed into the kidney and preferably down the ureter. If not, as much wire as possible is coiled within the kidney to provide maximum stability for dilatation.
- Secondly, as soon as possible, the creation of a universal guide wire (UGW).

Track Dilatation

Whether using Amplatz serial dilators, car aerial dilators, balloon or single-stage dilators, e.g. Webb SSD or "mini perc" dilators, they all involve the passage of at least one dilator from the skin into the renal collecting system.

Track Size

This varies depending on the proposed procedure:

- Routine stone fragmentation – 26 Fr
- "Mini Perc" < 20 Fr
- Large-volume staghorn calculus removal – 28–32 Fr
- Endoscopic pyeloplasty – 22–24 Fr
- Paediatric PCNL – 16 Fr

Track Dilatation

Aim

The aim of track dilatation is to insert the dilator and its sheath into the collecting system without kinking or dislodging the guide wire, or displacing the kidney.

Principles

- All dilators must be inserted under II screening.
- At all times, the direction of both the dilator and guide wire must be parallel to each other.

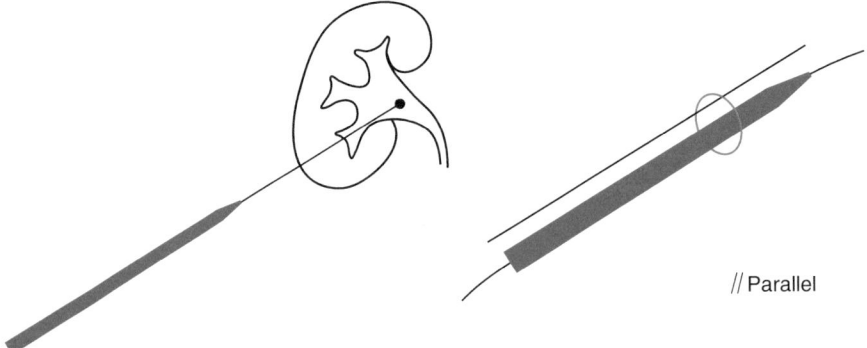

Fig. 5.1 Renal dilators must be inserted over and parallel to the path of guide wire

- Guide wire angulation can result in the following scenarios:
  - Kinked guide wire
  - Guide wire dislodged within or displaced from the kidney
  - Rotation, displacement or "flipping" of the kidney.

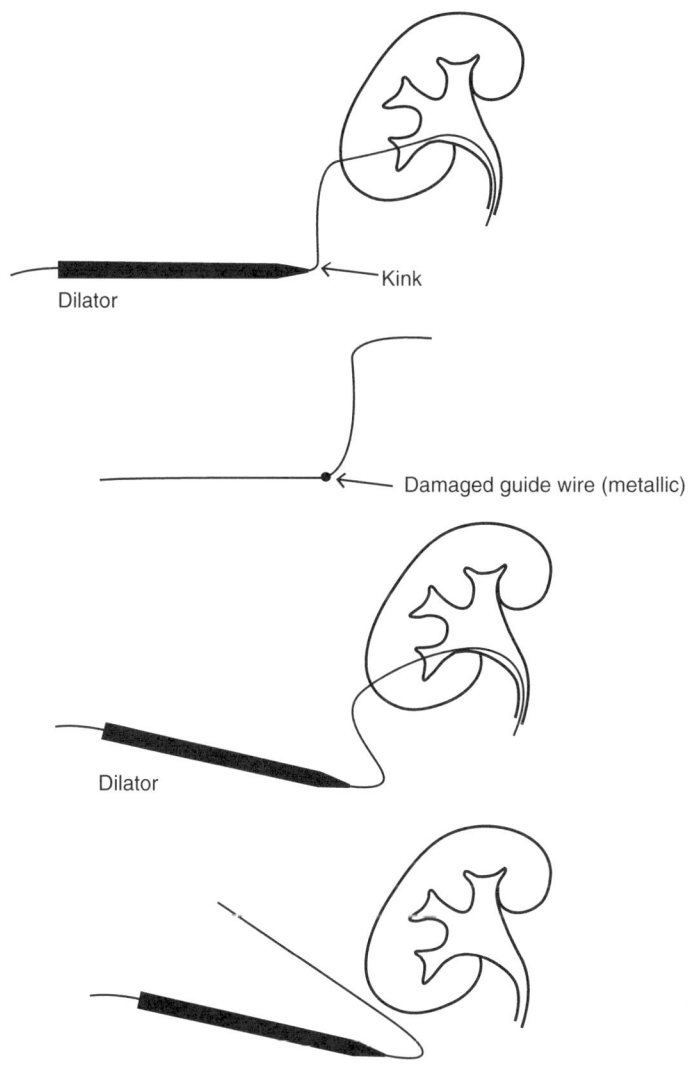

Fig. 5.2 If a dilator is passed at an angle to the guide wire, it will kink and may displace the guide wire

Fig. 5.3 Angled dilation over a guide wire, particularly with a lower pole puncture, can easily flip or rotate the kidney forwards

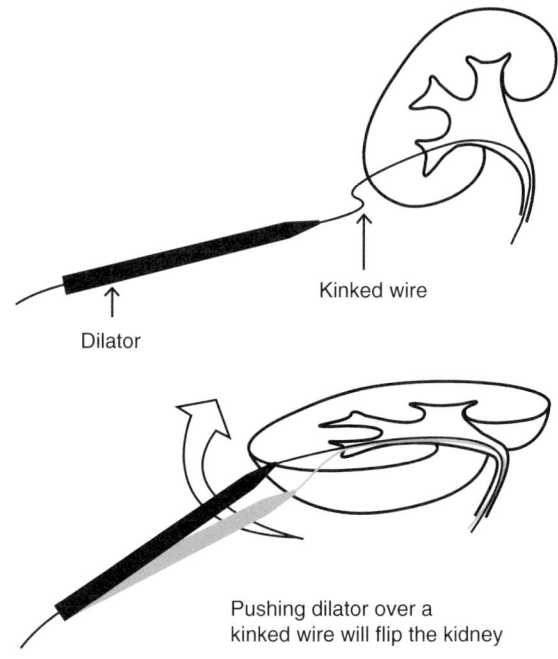

Kinked Guide Wire

- Once a metallic guide wire is kinked, it is useless and cannot be used for dilation.
- It must be removed.
- If the needle sheath can be threaded over the kink into the kidney, the guide wire can sometimes be replaced (this is an uncommon but occasionally lucky scenario, always worth a try)
- If not, the guide wire must be removed and a new puncture made.
- I use hydrophilic guide wires for all my punctures.
- This is because the inherent frictionless movement of the wire allows the wire to coil easily within the kidney or even better, to pass through the pelviureteric junction and smoothly down the ureter.
- Hydrophilic guide wires do not crush when held by artery forceps.
- Metallic guide wires are fragile and easily crush if grasped by artery forceps, rendering them useless.
- I use a metallic "J wire" as a retrieval wire when dealing with a "through and through" puncture.

The Body Wall Component of the Nephrostomy Track

- Once a guide wire is stable within the kidney, formal track dilatation may commence.
- The path to the kidney should be as frictionless as possible to allow tactile feedback during dilatation of the kidney.
- The major sites of friction are as follows:
  - Skin
  - Lumbodorsal fascia
  - Scar tissue from previous surgery

The Skin

Once the surgeon is confident that the guide wire is satisfactorily placed, the skin puncture should be extended by incising the skin and dermis with a scalpel either side of the guide wire, approximately 1 cm in length, parallel to Langer's lines. The scalpel must cut the full thickness of the dermis.

This will allow free movement of the dilator at the entry site.

Lumbodorsal Fascia

- I pass a pair of straight artery forceps under II control alongside the guide wire in the direction of the puncture, so the closed tips are just short of the kidney.
- It is clear to the surgeon when the tips traverse the lumbar dorsal fascia because there is a palpable "give".
- The forceps are then opened under II screening. The surgeon feels the lumbo dorsal fascia splitting and separating.
- The forceps are then relaxed, but not completely closed, as they may otherwise grasp and extract the guide wire. The forceps should be removed slowly, checking with II to ensure the wire has not been inadvertently grasped.
- This may seem quite a "physical method" of a track dilatation, but in over 30 years I have not had a complication from this manoeuvre.
- However, it should not be used for any supracostal puncture, as opening the forceps tips could tear the pleura.
- This technique also dilates and separates body wall scar tissue.
- At this stage, the track is prepared and the sites of potential friction cleared, so the dilator and Amplatz sheath may be introduced.

Track Dilation

In a routine adult stone case, I use a Webb Single-Stage dilator (26 Fr).

This dilator will usually pass easily into the kidney in a single passage. The diameter allows irrigation and free movement of a standard nephroscope.

As a result of the oval shape of nephroscopes, their widest dimension will be greater than the radius of a circular Amplatz sheath of the same French gauge. Hence the selection of a 26 Fr Amplatz sheath for a 22 Fr Nephroscope.

There can be significant resistance to the passage of a dilator, particularly if introduced between ribs, or at the level of the lumbo dorsal fascia, even when the fascia has been split with artery forceps.

This may result in a sudden "jerk" forwards as the dilator passes through one of these areas of resistance.

This "jerking" of the dilator tip may cause kinking and displacement of the guide wire or damage to the kidney. The surgeon must anticipate this potential hazard and avoid sudden over advancement of the dilator.

The surgeon is responsible for every step of a PCNL.

Guide Wire

The surgeon must control the guide wire, holding it with the non-dominant hand, so the guide wire does not become displaced during the dilatation.

Hydrophilic guide wires can easily slip or spring out if not carefully maintained. They should be grasped by artery forceps. These will not damage a hydrophilic guide wire.

Dilator

The surgeon must prevent uncontrolled movements, e.g. jerking, or over advancement of the dilator and prevent angulation, which may lead to displacement of the guide wire.

The below diagram outlines the dilation technique. The surgeon maintains the guide wire (hydrophilic) with artery forceps using the non-dominant hand. The dominant or dilating hand rests on the patient's back on the ulnar aspect, with the thumb, index and middle finger free to rotate and advance the dilator, holding the dilator in the classical "pencil grip".

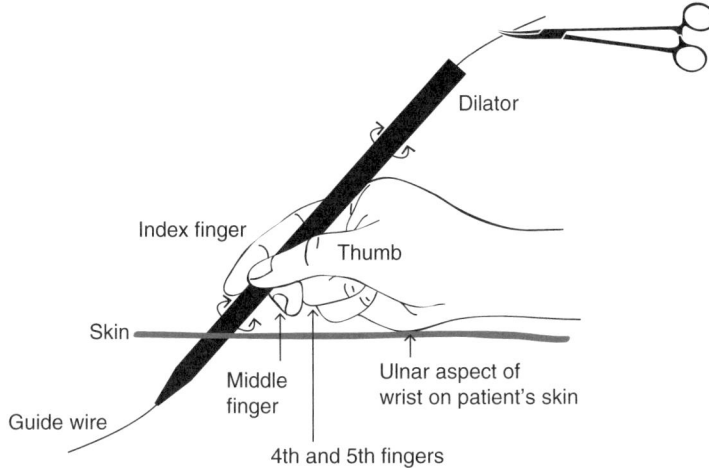

Fig. 5.4 Safe technique of passing a dilator over the guide wire

The dilator is advanced and rotated simultaneously. This allows the tip of the dilator to gently enter and dilate the renal substance and capsule and decreases friction from skin and fascial layers on the dilator as it advances.

Commencement of the Track and Kidney Dilation

The guide wire is grasped and held externally by the surgeon at the outer end of the dilator using artery forceps.

If the wire is not held close to the dilator, it may spring out. This is a tedious but avoidable scenario.

The dilator is inserted parallel to the direction of the original scalpel stab, needle track and guide wire.

The dilating hand is placed, ulnar side down, on the patient and the dilator controlled by the thumb, index and middle fingers using the "pencil grip".

The tip of the dilator is gently rotated and advanced through the skin after the skin puncture has been enlarged using the scalpel.

II monitoring confirms that the direction of dilator and the wire are parallel. If not, the course of the dilator must be realigned under II screening.

Retrograde contrast should be infused gently through the retrograde ureteric catheter via minimal volume extension tubing. Vigorous infusion can result in pyelovenous and forniceal extravasation of contrast, resulting in radiological obliteration of the collecting system. A gentle infusion will delineate and distend the targeted calyx.

The dilator is slowly and gently advanced towards the kidney, rotating and screening throughout.

The introduction of the tip of the dilator into the kidney is monitored by II.

If the dilator is displacing the kidney, or not entering easily, the dilator should be removed and exchanged for a 12 or 14 Fr fascial dilator. These smaller dilators will "drill" rather than separate the renal capsule and parenchyma without displacing the kidney (this manoeuvre is only occasionally required).

This initial "drill" opens the track sufficiently for the entry of the tip of the SSD. At this stage, the SSD can be reintroduced. Once the shoulder of the SSD dilator is within the collecting system, an Amplatz sheath is placed over the dilator and inserted by simultaneous advancement and rotation.

While rotating and advancing the Amplatz sheath, the dilator must be stabilised to prevent it being inadvertently over-advanced into the kidney.

To do this, the surgeon holds the external end of the dilator with his non-dominant hand, with his elbow firmly on the patient's back. By doing so, the dilator is safely fixed.

Care must be taken not to advance the leading edge of the Amplatz dilator past the shoulder of the dilator. The edge of the Amplatz sheath is bevelled, oblique and sharp and if not directly applied to the shaft of the dilator, can cut parenchyma, collecting system and vessels.

When using the Webb Single-Stage Dilator, a proximal external marker on the dilator notifies the surgeon when the leading tip of the Amplatz sheath is at the shoulder of the dilator.

With all dilating systems, the passage of the Amplatz sheath over the dilator into the kidney must be monitored by II.

Once the Amplatz sheath is safely inside the kidney, the following should be done:

- The dilator may be removed.
- The guide wire must be re-grasped at the outer edge of the Amplatz sheath with forceps. The assistant now maintains this wire.
- The Amplatz sheath must also be supported by the assistant, but NOT PUSHED IN, a common mistake made by assistants in the mistaken belief they are being helpful. Advancing the Amplatz sheath without a dilator may result in severe trauma to the parenchyma, vessels and collecting system.

The kidney is now ready for nephroscopy.

Nephroscopy and Stone Removal

Plan

Every PCNL is unique.

The surgeon must have specific aims, a "game plan" and a "fall back plan" before commencing any PCNL, anticipating potential difficulties and complications.

In the case of an infection-related calculus, the aim is complete clearance of all stone.

If the stone is very large, the surgeon may plan for multiple punctures, followed by elective ESWL or "second look" PCNL.

If the stone is large, complex, infected and/or associated with a urinary diversion, it may not be possible, safe or practicable to clear all the stone, even by multiple operations. Many of these patients are high medical risk and medically unfit for repeated anaesthetics or anatomically unsuitable for ESWL or secondary PCNL approaches, so the surgeon has "only one opportunity" to remove as much stone as possible. These patients usually remain infected in any event, and tend to represent with stone recurrences in spite of initial complete stone clearance.

In this scenario, I aim for "stone palliation". The primary aim of the PCNL is to remove all obstructing (pelvic or calyceal) stones first, and then as much of the bulk of the stone mass that is safely accessible within 2 hours of nephroscopy.

It is well documented that continuing a PCNL in excess of two hours is associated with a significant increase in all PCNL morbidities. This "philosophy" of "stone palliation" can be applied equally to recurring metabolic calculi, especially cystine, and those in horseshoe kidneys or associated with neurogenic bladders.

This concept of "stone palliation" is important to discuss and fully explain to a patient with recurring stones, and their physicians.

Both the patient and the surgeon must accept that it is not practical or safe to attempt to completely clear every kidney of all stone, and that the primary aim of PCNL is to unobstruct and preserve the kidney.

Nephroscopes

The majority of PCNLs are performed using rigid nephroscopes.

Flexible nephroscopes have limited applications. They can be useful as a delayed secondary procedure following an extensive PCNL or ESWL, to electively clear residual fragments. It is often written that flexible nephroscopy may access difficult calyces during an extended PCNL. This has not been my experience, as once well into a large PCNL, there is usually bleeding and the inaccessible calyces are usually quite angled with respect to the existing track. The flexible scope is limited by reduced irrigation due to a narrow channel, and compromised tip deflection within the small confines and acutely angled anatomy of the kidney. In my experience, the optimal application of the flexible nephroscopy (and holmium laser) is to reach and clear the medial stone bulk in a horseshoe kidney. In this case, the course is only slightly curved, so the length and lesser angulation required to reach these stones is ideally suited to flexible nephrolithotripsy.

Flexible nephroscopy can also be very useful during "mini-PCNL" which is virtually bloodless. One needs to upsize to the longer 21/24 Fr sheath and maintain the sheath lumen in the renal pelvis. This allows the flexed tip to access the calyceal necks and avoid the curved nephroscope to catch on and be damaged by the sheath tip.

The rigid nephroscope has an offset eye piece. The lens may be set at a right angle to the shaft of the endoscope, the "crank handle" or oblique at 30° the "angled".

Either type of offset lens allows the passage of rigid lithotrites and surgical instruments directly through the working channel of the nephroscope. The combination of camera and an offset lens can be disorientating for the surgeon.

This special orientation of the camera must remain constant. The nephroscope should move within its attachment independent to the camera. The surgeon's hand must maintain the camera in a constant orientation. This connection between the surgeon's hand and the camera becomes the urologists "cerebellum".

By keeping the camera orientation fixed, all movements of the nephroscope and the instruments through the nephroscope are instinctively orientated.

I do this by holding the camera and the cable, which always exits the camera at 6 o'clock, in my left or non-dominant hand. All instrumentation is by my right hand. This combination gives me completely accurate spatial orientation throughout the PCNL.

Most nephroscopes have a foroblique lens, varying between 10° and 30°. In other words, their view is angled, not directly ahead.

The instrument channels are eccentric, not central.

Therefore rotation of the nephroscope will provide a wide field of vision, resulting in good access to the majority of the collecting system, except for "parallel lie" and obliquely offset calyces.

Surgeons should be comfortable and facile with the capacity and limitations of their preferred nephroscope.

Blood Clots

Blood clots are the bane of percutaneous renal surgery!

There is no optimal solution for their removal.

The renal pelvis and calyces are a small non-distensible system, so barbotage, which is so effective in the bladder, does not work well within the kidney, and can result in extravasation of fluid or collapse of the collecting system.

Similarly, suction will not aspirate clots, but it will collapse the renal pelvis obscuring vision.

The optimal method of managing blood clots is to avoid them by:

(a) Uncomplicated percutaneous renal puncture.
(b) Maintaining the Amplatz sheath within the collecting system (should the sheath retract, the parenchyma, which is tamponaded by the sheath, will usually bleed).
(c) Continuously irrigating, even when changing instruments.
(d) Always having two irrigation bags open and running, each hanging at a different level and ensuring that your technicians are monitoring these. Intervals of no irrigation must be avoided, or clot rapidly develops.
(e) Inserting the nephroscope into the Amplatz sheath and continue irrigation during instrument changes. This is very important. It is very frustrating to look back into what was a crystal clear renal pelvis to find it full of clot.

(f) Using the 'mini-PCNL' instruments in my opinion causes far less bleeding than conventional PCNL.

Even though the operative field may appear clear during endoscopy, as with a TUR Prostate, profuse venous bleeding can occur in the absence of irrigation.

Unfortunately, blood clots still form.

Clots are occasionally helpful for the clearance of small stone fragments. Gentle extraction of a clot as an intact entity containing calculi can function as a "coagulum pyelolithotomy".

Clot Removal

The most efficient method of removal in my experience is to very gently and slowly lift the clot out of the sheath with alligator stone forceps.

Alligator forceps are marginally better than triradiates, but both are poor, as they crush and break fresh clots.

There are no effective "clot extractors" because clots are so friable and fragile.

Suckers are of little help, as the small collecting system does not distend and rapidly collapses.

Painstaking clearance of clots is essential before proceeding with the nephrolithotomy.

Clots can mask stone fragments and guide wires. Insertion of graspers blindly into a clot is dangerous and may result in inadvertent grasping of a guide wire and accidentally removing it, or grasping, tearing or perforating the renal pelvis.

Universal Guide Wire

The establishment of a universal guide wire (UGW) is my first aim in all PCNLs.

A UGW traverses the collecting system from the skin to the urethral meatus.

The UGW is fixed at either end with artery forceps. Once a UGW is established, operative access is improved and the kidney aligns with the direction of the puncture, even if it has been initially displaced. Dilatation is easier and safer and nephrostomy insertion and antegrade stent placement is facilitated. No matter how much

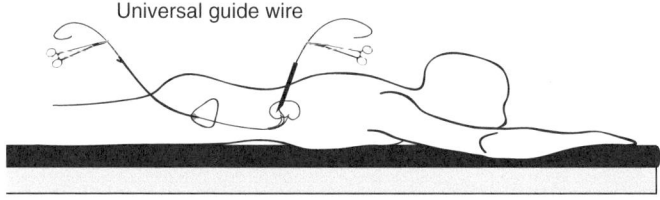

Fig. 5.5 The universal guide wire, running from the external tip of the ureteric catheter and, exiting the Amplatz sheath, fixed by artery forceps at either end

bleeding or trauma to the kidney or collecting system occurs, a UGW will always enable the surgeon to recover the situation and safely gain access to the renal pelvis and establish a nephrostomy.

The Creation of a Universal Guide Wire

The first step is to visualise the renal pelvis.

The assistant then passes the floppy end of a straight hydrophilic guide wire from the bladder through the ureteric catheter, which has previously been brought through the craniofacial drape when the patient is prepared in the prone position.

The surgeon visualises the guide wire as it exits the ureteric catheter into the renal pelvis, and grasps it with alligator or triradiate forceps.

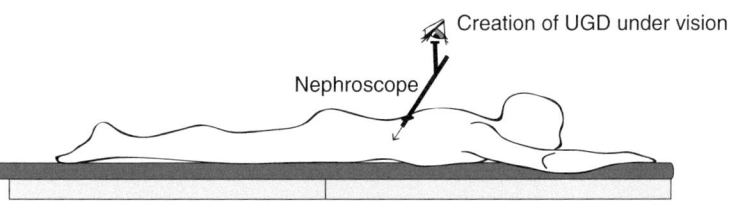

Fig. 5.6 Creation of a UGW – first step/nephroscopy

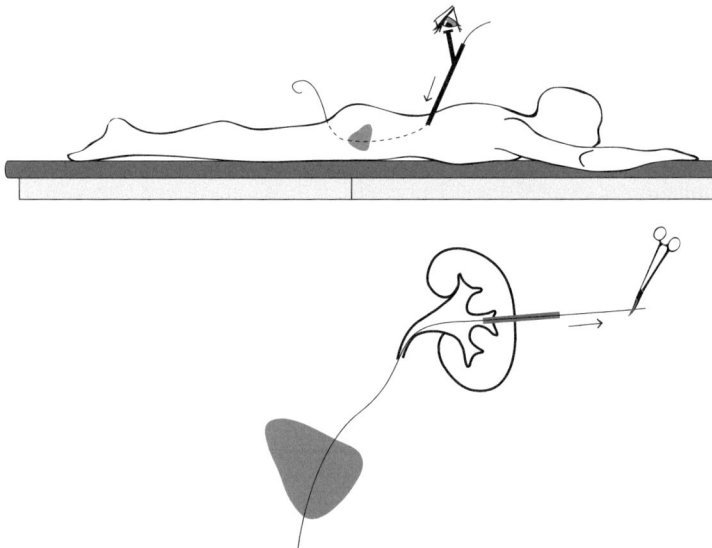

Fig. 5.7 Creation of UGW. While the surgeon looks into the renal pelvis, the assistant passes a hydrophilic guide wire through the outer end of the RGC

The assistant then feeds the wire towards the surgeon through the ureteric catheter. As the wire is fed upwards, the surgeon extracts the floppy end of the guide wire out through the Amplatz sheath.

Artery forceps are then applied to the guide wire at the proximal and distal ends. These artery forceps must then be separately attached to the patient drapes to prevent displacement.

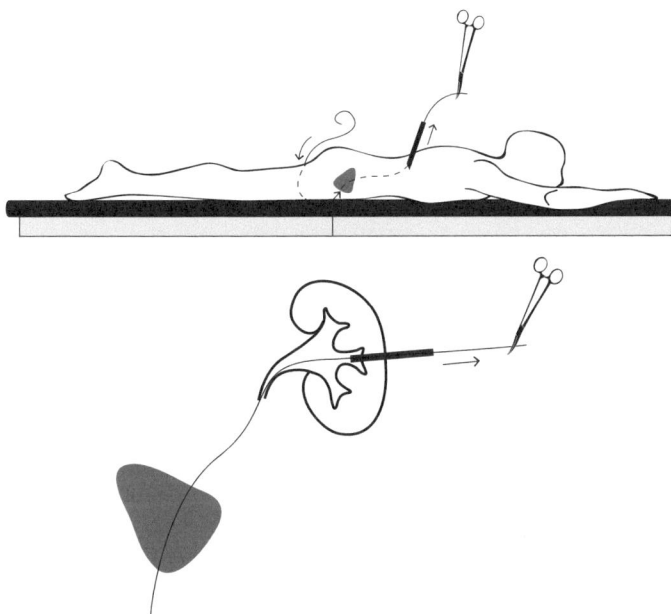

Fig. 5.8 Creation of UGW. The guide wire is extracted from the kidney by the surgeon through the Amplatz sheath

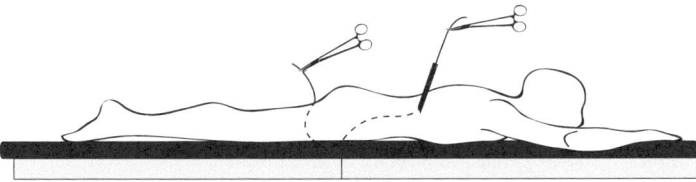

Fig. 5.9 Creation of UGW. Once the guide wire exits the Amplatz sheath, both ends of the UGW are clamped by forceps, which in turn are separately fixed to the drapes.

Advantages of a Universal Guide Wire

With a UGW in place, the surgeon can always re-enter the kidney to perform nephroscopy, place a nephrostomy or antegrade stent, or introduce larger dilators.

In 'Mini-PCNL', a UGW allows the surgeon to safely re-introduce the operating sheath alongside the UGW. The wireless sheath functions more effectively with respect to flow and the 'vacuum cleaner' extraction of stone fragments. The sheath also exhibits increased versatility of movement and access within the renal collecting system.

No matter what complications occur, even in the event of significant tearing of the collecting system, the surgeon cannot lose the nephrostomy track. The UGW cannot migrate outside the collecting system.

Routine dilatation of a PCNL track tends to displace and angulate the kidney forwards and medially and so develop an angle between the pelvis and ureter.

The UGW straightens the nephrostomy track and directly orientates the kidney along the axis of the wire for subsequent endoscopy or dilation. I find nephroscopy is much easier and direct once the UGW is established.

The UGW stabilises the kidney, which can be extremely useful for subsequent Target or "Y punctures".

With an established UGW, large dilators, up to 32 and 34 Fr can be introduced without fear of the displacement of the kidney or damage to the renal pelvis, as the UGW is fixed within the lumen of the ureter.

The UGW traverses a gentle curve and so facilitates access to the pelviureteric junction and upper ureter. This is particularly useful for antegrade ureteroscopy and percutaneous endopyelotomy.

The UGW facilitates easy antegrade placement of a double J stent from the kidney to the bladder. This can be particularly useful during endoscopic pyeloplasty or insertion of a stent into an ileal conduit. It is not always possible to manipulate a stent through the vesicoureteric junction into the bladder using an antegrade approach or through a nephroscope over a guide wire coiled in the bladder. It is much easier over a straightened and tensioned UGW.

A UGW also facilitates synchronous conduitoscopy. A guide wire can be inserted from the kidney, into the conduit, where it is grasped from below with a flexible endoscope to create a UGW.

During percutaneous endopyelotomy, the UGW straightens and fixes the direction for the urethrotome. By placing a second guide wire antegrade alongside the UGW into the ureter through the urethrotome, the phenomenon of "bow stringing displacement" of the original guide wire is prevented.

When extracting calculi percutaneously from the upper ureter, the ureter tends to migrate medially and angulate on introduction of the nephroscope. This makes antegrade ureteroscopy difficult and sometimes impossible. This mucosal angle can also catch the edge of the stone on the ureteric mucosa as they are extracted from the ureter by basket or grasper. With gentle traction on the UGW from above and below, this angle will straighten.

Stone Fragmentation

Two standard rigid lithotrites are in common use.
They both fragment stones by a "Jack Hammer" effect, but differ in their energy sources:

1. Ultrasound or piezoelectric vibration – the Sonotrode
2. Pneaumatic or ballistic – the "Lithoclast" and other brands

Alternative Energy Sources for Stone Fragmentation

- Laser – Although newer laser systems are capable of fragmenting large hard calculi, I prefer to reserve laser lithotripsy for flexible nephroscopy (particularly for clearing calculi in a horseshoe kidney) or 'Mini-PCNL' in which 'stone dusting' is most suitable. I find it difficult to justify the high cost of a disposable fiber in cases where the re-usable lithoclast probe is just as fast, safe, and effective.
- Electrohydraulic – these bipolar cables create a shockwave by passing a current between electrodes at the tip of a flexible wire. They can damage the nephroscope, fragment the lens and cause bleeding and perforation of tissues. It is now rare for electrohydraulic probes to be used for PCNL or ureteroscopy since the introduction of rigid and laser lithotrites.

Optimal Lithotrites for Stone Fragmentations

The "optimal lithotrite" for a PCNL is a combination of ultrasonic and pneaumatic instruments. They can be used in combination, or separately, depending on the stone mass, size, composition, hardness and location. Laser lithotripsy is confined to flexible nephroscopes or the fine bone "mini perc" nephroscopes.

Aims of Stone Fragmentation

The surgeon's aim is to reduce large stones to smaller fragments that can be easily and safely extracted or aspirated. Reducing stones to large fragments is faster and associated with decreased blood loss and less dispersion of stone fragments throughout the kidney and down the ureter. Larger stone fragments are easier to find endoscopically and radiologically.

It is not always possible to physically extract stone fragments with grasping forceps. For instance, stones in calyceal diverticula, tightly applied calyces or calculi impacted in the upper ureter. In these situations, "drilling and aspiration" using a sonotrode is superior. Stone 'dusting' where the calculus is reduced to very fine particles which flush out, is very applicable to Mini PCNL.

The Sonotrode

This is a hollow metal tube that transmits vibrations generated by a piezoelectric crystal proximally. The probe drills stones to create small sandy particles of about 2 mm diameter, which are aspirated. It can also be used to fragment or reduce large stones into smaller pieces that can be removed with graspers.

The vibrations cause extreme and rapid heating of the probe. To avoid overheating, the sonotrode requires continuous and uninterrupted irrigation to maintain cooling and clear vision. The aspirations also suck small sandy stone particles out through the lumen of the sonotrode.

The vibrations of the sonotrode do not damage tissues or endoscopes provided that the probe does not overheat.

The sonotrode is particularly suited to softer stones such as struvite and calcium oxalate. It is also very effective for the fragmentation of cystine calculi, as long as they are not heavily calcified.

Because the sonotrode aspirates small stone particles simultaneously, it does not need to be repeatedly removed and reintroduced.

As a result, the sonotrode is optimal for treating stones in confined spaces or cavities, such as when beginning to obtain access to the collecting system in which a staghorn calculus completely occupies the collecting system. Other situations where the sonotrode is optimal include stones that are a complete cast of a calyx, calculi in a calyceal diverticulum or an impacted pelviureteric junction or upper ureteric stone.

As the sonotrode does not need to be removed during stone destruction, it is particularly useful where the track is tenuous (e.g., a calyceal diverticulum where there is little guide wire in the kidney).

The sonotrode is reusable.

The sonotrode cannot be used in the lower ureter, as it is too large.

The sonotrode does not fragment extremely hard calculi.

The sonotrode can be particularly slow or inadequate for clearing large staghorn calculi.

Constant irrigation is required. Despite the sophistication of the sonotrodes, most systems have complicated pumps and suction mechanisms, which can be difficult to set up, malfunction and the fluid aspiration often causes collapse of the renal pelvis, all generating stress amongst the theatre technicians and surgeons.

To be effective, the sonotrode must be directly applied to the calculus with some pressure. This is not a problem for impacted stones, but can result in stone migration in the renal pelvis.

Choice of Lithotrite

The size, nature, structure and anatomical disposition of the stone will all influence the choice of lithotrite deployed.

Ultrasonic Lithotrite (Sonotrode)

Optimal indications:

- Struvite calculi.
- Cystine calculi (non-calcified).
- Impacted stones, e.g. large stones in the ureter, calyceal diverticulum or calyx.
- Multiple small stones.
- To enter a kidney where there is limited space, using the sonotrode to excavate a cavity to provide room for the introduction of the dilator and Amplatz sheath, e.g. large staghorn calculus or calyceal diverticulum.

Pneaumatic Lithoclast

This has replaced electrohydraulic probes for the fragmentation of large, hard calculi.

The pneaumatic lithoclast fragments stones by a simple jackhammer mechanism.

The probe is cheap, safe, breaks all hard stones and is fast and reusable. It is also excellent in the bladder and ureter, and has fine probes suitable for the "Mini Perc" nephroscopes.

The pneaumatic lithoclast does not become hot.

There are limitations to the pneaumatic lithoclast. Firstly, it does not aspirate calculi. The lithoclast only fragments stones. As a result, the stone fragments it creates must be physically extracted. This requires repeated interchanges of the lithotrite, grasping forceps and nephroscope.

During these interchanges, bleeding, track loss and stone migration may occur.

The lithoclast is difficult to use in confined spaces, because it does not aspirate fragments or create room for grasping stones. However, it is possible to perform 'stone-dusting' on some calculi using the lithoclast.

Therefore, in the initial approach to a large calculus, the surgeon will often use a sonotrode to primarily excavate a cavity into a calyx. This facilitates the introduction of the nephroscope and Amplatz sheath, and the surgeon has the option to convert to the lithoclast, which is more efficient in a larger space through a stable Amplatz sheath.

To fragment a stone using a lithoclast, the calculus must be immobilised.

As fragmentation requires the lithoclast probe to be applied directly to the calculus, stone fragments can be propelled forwards and so migrate into calyces or along the ureter.

Summary

It is essential that a surgeon has access to both pneumatic and ultrasonic lithotrites at least and is thoroughly familiar with the optimal application of these devices, their advantages and disadvantages and relative indications, depending on the stone and renal anatomy. If performing 'Mini-PCNL' or flexible nephroscopy, laser lithotripsy should also be available and familiar to the surgeon and staff.

Stone Extraction for PCNL

Instruments

- Alligator forceps
- Triradiate forceps
- Others – e.g., ureteric baskets

Alligator Forceps

Alligator forceps have rigid hinged jaws, smooth rounded atraumatic tips and a hinged handle, which grasps stones by a forward closure.

The jaws open without advancement of the forceps and are safe in the upper ureter and calyces.

By virtue of the hinge, they are expensive and fragile and prone to breakage if larger stones are firmly grasped.

Even though the thin jaws will cut through clot, they remain the optimal instrument for removing clots, although still inefficient.

Alligator forceps cannot grasp large stone fragments.

As the jaws close by advancement, they push larger stones away.

Alligator forceps can be used in confined spaces and are efficient for the removal of small stone particles.

Fig. 5.10 Grasping a calculus with the alligator forceps. The jaws are hinged, so they open directly under vision

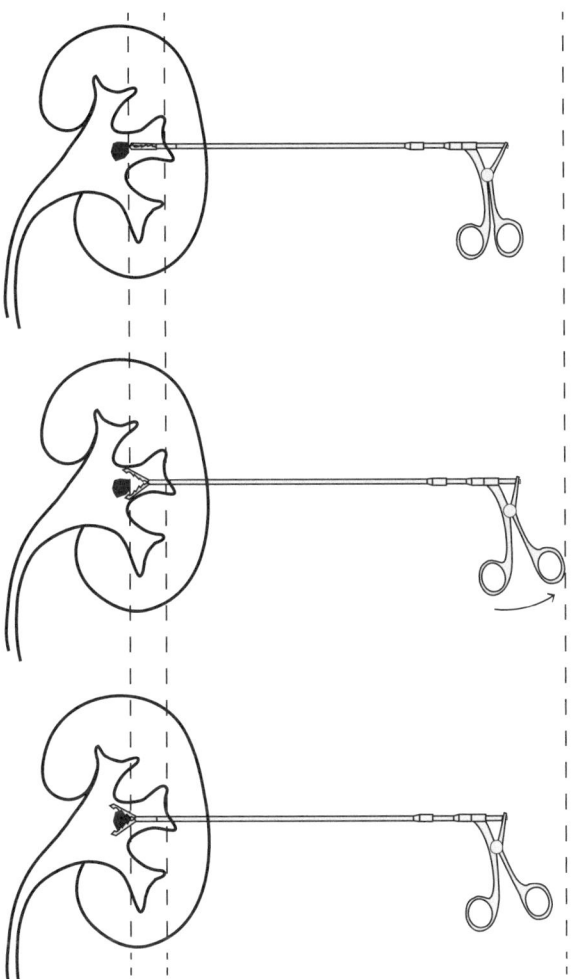

Triradiate Forceps

Triradiate forceps have no hinges or jaws. Grasping is effected by sharp angulated retro pointing metal tines.

Triradiate forceps are rigid, cheap, strong, long lasting, durable and can grasp and extract larger stone fragments.

The tines have to extend distally from the shaft of the instrument to open. This requires the nephroscope and the barrel of the forceps to be retracted to permit the jaws to advance. As a result, they can be inefficient and even impossible to open in a confined space such as calyceal diverticulum, tight calyx or ureter.

Fig. 5.11 Grasping a stone with triradiate forceps. As the tines move forward to grasp a stone, the forceps need to be retracted

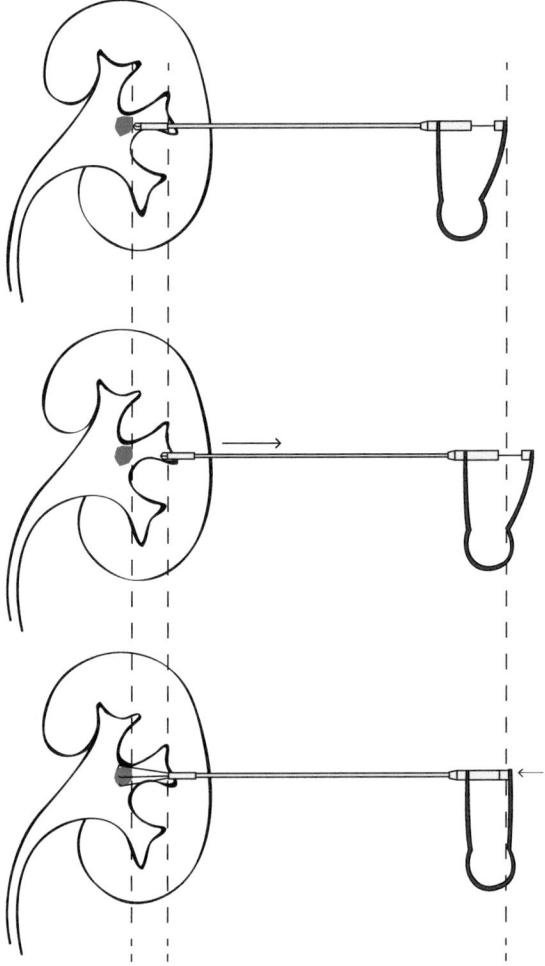

The sharp tines easily perforate and tear the collecting system. They must only be deployed under vision in an open space to ensure they do not pierce the renal pelvis or the ureteric wall.

The optimal application of triradiate forceps is to extract larger stone fragments in the renal pelvis or a dilated calyx.

Baskets

Standard ureteric baskets are of limited value in the kidney, unless used through a flexible nephroscope.

Older stone baskets were spiral in shape and designed for use in the ureter, where the calculus is usually immobilised, preventing the stone springing out as the basket closes. This is often the case when spiral baskets are deployed in cavities such as the bladder or renal pelvis.

If using a basket in the kidney, select one of the new tipless ureteric baskets that has a rounded, smooth tip. They are much more effective in calyces and the renal pelvis, particularly in combination with a flexible nephroscope. I find it ideal for stone extraction during 'Mini-PCNL' if the fragments cannot be cleared by the 'vacuum cleaner effect'.

Summary

It is essential for the surgeon to have both triradiate and alligator graspers.

Triradiates are ideal for the fast and safe removal of large stone fragments in an open operating space such as in the renal pelvis.

Alligator forceps are superior for the removal of small fragments, stones in confined spaces, and are safe in the ureter and calyces.

Stone Clearance

Although the aim of all PCNL operations is complete stone clearance, this is not always possible with a single PCNL.

The surgeon must estimate and plan the degree of clearance and discuss the potential outcome with the patient prior to surgery.

Most stone cases fall into the following scenarios:

1. Complete stone clearance

    Complete stone clearance is optimal for infection-related calculi, stones in a calyceal diverticulum or those in poorly draining calyces that are unsuitable for secondary ESWL, particularly within a lower pole calyx with a long thin infundibulum.

2. Elective combination therapy

    The typical scenario for combined therapy (where complete clearance is desired, but preoperative evaluation suggests this is unlikely to be achieved by a single PCNL, e.g., multiple PCNLs or PCNL plus ESWL) is where there is a large and complex distribution of stones, with a bulky central stone and multiple peripheral extensions, which require more than two or three punctures for clearance.

    A PCNL should not continue for more than 2 h. With a complex and large stone mass, the surgeon should plan for elective repeat PCNL, ESWL or FURS.

3. "Palliative" PCNL – stone control

    There are recurrent stone formers, particularly those with urinary diversions, neuropathic bladders, poorly controlled cystinuria and horseshoe kidneys in whom no matter how well the stone is primarily treated, regular recurrences will occur.

The aim of treatment in these scenarios is elective, safe, debulking of the stone and unobstruction of the remainder of the collecting system with the least potential damage to the kidney.

This "concept" of "palliative" stone management must be clearly explained to patients (and their physicians) before surgery.

Assessment of Stone Clearance at PCNL

Two intraoperative modalities are available to the surgeon. Both should be employed in every case, to assess the degree of stone clearance:

(a) Complete endoscopic surveillance of the collecting system with the nephroscope prior to II.
(b) II screening once the kidney appears endoscopically clear.

It is important to compare the final images to the stored image saved at the time of the initial renal puncture prior to contrast infusion.

Often, the II will suggest there is a stone in a narrow calyx that was initially empty. This is often contrast and not a stone. This artefact will usually clear with a saline flush.

Nephrostomy Post PCNL

I believe the function of a nephrostomy is to drain urine. I do not believe they are efficient at draining blood clots or stone fragments.

Furthermore, I have not been convinced that a large nephrostomy will tamponade bleeding. In fact, as with other renal trauma, if the urine is drained and the renal parenchyma is allowed to return to his normal anatomy (similar to the management of blunt renal trauma), unless major arterial trauma is present, bleeding (which is usually venous) will settle conservatively. It follows that bleeding is more likely to be prolonged in a kidney in which a large tube or balloon separates and holds the renal parenchyma apart, preventing natural tamponade.

Nephrostomy Types

- "Cope" loop nephrostomy
- Foley balloon catheter nephrostomies
- Tube (splinted)
- "Tubeless" – an internal antegrade JJ stent without external nephrostomy drainage

"Cope" Loop Nephrostomy

These are cheap, readily available and can be found in all radiological and operating suites.

They are soft, tubular and 10–12 Fr in circumference. They are easy to insert over either a guide wire or an obturator through the Amplatz sheath.

They drain urine well.

They have small drainage holes, which do not become blocked by clot.

Being fine bore and soft, they are comfortable, move easily with respiration and so do not traumatise or flip out of the kidney with patient movement.

The "Cope" loop is ideal for an antegrade nephrostogram.

The "Cope" nephrostomy facilitates the easy insertion of a guide wire for antegrade basketing of calculi, double J stent insertion or a secondary PCNL.

It is important for the nursing staff to be familiar with the externally tied retaining string that maintains the Cope loop.

It is also essential to be aware that removal of a "Cope" loop nephrostomy in the presence of a double J stent commonly results in the double J stent being inadvertently extracted synchronously.

Where a double J stent or a "Cope" loop nephrostomy is present together, the nephrostomy should only be removed in the radiology department over a guide wire under fluoroscopy, never on the ward.

Foley Catheter

I do not use this type of nephrostomy. I find they are large, bulky, uncomfortable and very difficult to remove if the balloon does not deflate. In the small confines of the renal pelvis, the single end hole is easily covered and obstructed.

I have not found that inflation of a Foley catheter balloon in the renal pelvis will tamponade significant bleeding.

Tube Nephrostomy (Splinted)

Early nephrostomies were simple tubes. These were impractical as they were uncomfortable and fell out of the kidney with respiratory movement. The tube could be maintained in position by splinting by an internal ureteric catheter, which went through the lumen of the nephrostomy and down the ureter, allowing the nephrostomy to move with the kidney without displacement. However, they were still less comfortable than the smaller and softer self-retaining nephrostomies. The splinted tube still has a place following significant pelvic injury.

Tubeless Nephrostomy

The insertion of a double J stent without a nephrostomy tube is advantageous following transpleural supracostal punctures, as no tube remains that traverses the pleural space.

I always use a tubeless nephrostomy following percutaneous endopyelotomy, as the patient requires a stent for 6 weeks following surgery anyway.

In a complicated PCNL where the track is lost, a tubeless nephrostomy can be created from above if a UGW has been established, or cystoscopically from below. This can be supplemented by insertion of a Yeates drain or Penrose Drain Tube into the nephrostomy track via the skin incision, as one would do at open renal surgery.

Technique of "Cope" Nephrostomy Insertion Following PCNL

Following PCNL, the renal pelvis and calyces are assessed endoscopically and radiologically.

With an Amplatz sheath in place, it is difficult to perform an accurate nephrostogram, because the contrast preferentially flows out of the Amplatz sheath. This can be overcome by inserting the appropriate dilator (the Webb dilator has a fine lumen) into the Amplatz sheath.

Attach the clear outer sheath of the renal puncture needle to a 20 cc syringe of contrast.

Insert the needle sheath into the lumen of the renal dilator so that it is "watertight" at the outer end. Under screening, infuse the contrast. As the contrast cannot now escape between the Amplatz sheath and the dilator, this produces an excellent nephrostogram.

The same can be performed using a Mini-PCNL SSD.

If the pelvis is accommodating, the "Cope" nephrostomy and trocar can be inserted through the Amplatz sheath, and the trocar removed during II screening.

Following confirmation that the nephrostomy is in the pelvis, the loop can be formed by tightening the string externally and fixing it below the Leur lock and rolling the external rubber sheath over the string.

This maintains the retaining loop and prevents leakage from the nephrostomy tube at the external string exit.

Contrast is then injected through the "Cope" to confirm that it is in correct position.

Once confirmed, either side of the Amplatz sheath can be cut with scissors parallel to its axis, and removed using the "peel away technique". This procedure splits the Amplatz sheath, pulling it apart using artery forceps gripping either side of the sheath. The split sheath easily extrudes from the patient without interfering with the nephrostomy.

Following the removal of the Amplatz sheath, I perform a second nephrostogram to confirm that the "Cope" loop remains well positioned within the kidney. If so, I remove the UGW and ureteric catheter and suture the "Cope" nephrostomy to the

Alternative Method of Insertion of the "Cope" Loop Nephrostomy

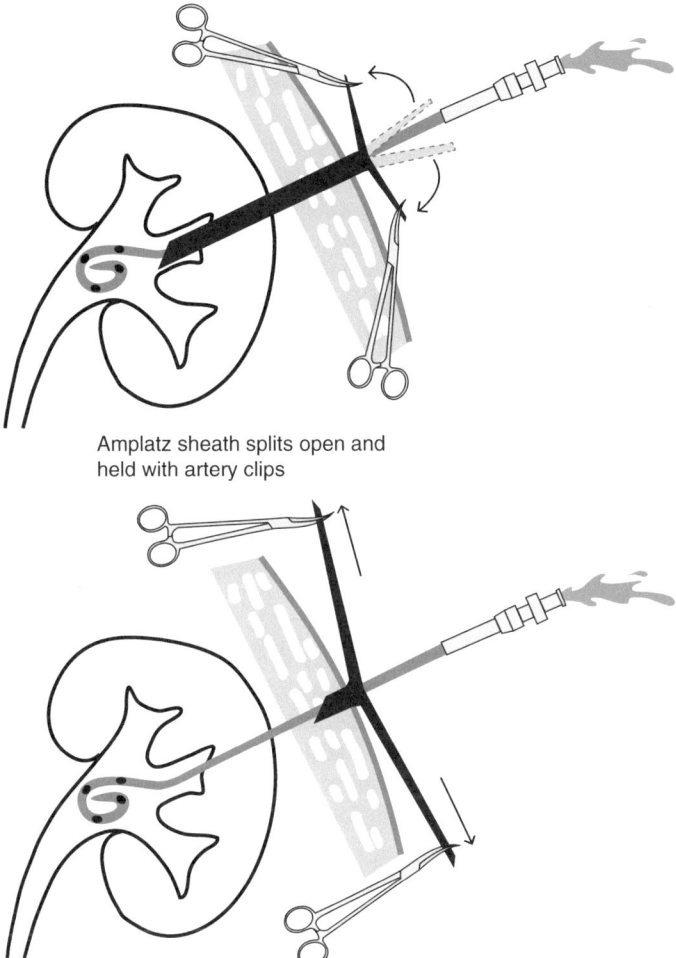

Fig. 5.12 Removal of the Amplatz sheath after inserting a nephrostomy by the "peel away" technique

skin using heavy silk suture and leaving a 1–2 cm "mesentry". The skin suture is loose, so the nephrostomy stab can still allow fluid to drain around the Cope tubing.

Alternative Method of Insertion of the "Cope" Loop Nephrostomy

Should the pelvis appear small, or in the case of a pelvic perforation, a second antegrade guide wire can be passed under vision alongside the UGW into the upper ureter.

The UGW is left as a backup if subsequent nephrostomy insertion fails.

The obturator is removed from the "Cope" nephrostomy and the tip of the Cope nephrostomy is threaded over the guide wire, into the renal pelvis monitored by II screening.

When screening confirms that the loop is at the level of the renal pelvis, the guide wire can be removed slowly, at the same time rotating the "Cope" nephrostomy between the thumb and forefinger. This manoeuvre encourages a loop to form without pulling on the string (if there is a renal pelvic laceration and the string is forcibly pulled, the "Cope" loop may extrude and form outside the perforation).

Once the loop has formed, the string can be tightened and fixed proximally.

Position is then confirmed by a nephrostogram.

In spite of this, the "Cope" can migrate outside the collecting system. If this occurs, the procedure can be repeated, but this time using the UGW to position the "Cope" nephrostomy loop. The UGW is always inside the lumen of the collecting system.

Lost Nephrostomy

If, for reasons such as trauma or tearing, or if the track is lost, and it is not possible to place a nephrostomy into the kidney even in the presence of a UGW, I insert a penrose drain tube on my finger tip along the PCNL track to the depth of the kidney and suture it to the skin. Alternatively, a Yeates drain or round tube can be inserted.

This creates the same perirenal drainage as used following open kidney surgery. This can be augmented by cystoscopic double J stent insertion if concerned.

Suturing the "Cope" Nephrostomy Tube to the Skin

The kidney and body wall move, often in opposite directions. This differential movement is magnified in obese patients.

A nephrostomy attached tightly to the skin

- Can be uncomfortable due to traction on the kidney, which is exacerbated during respiration.
- May be pulled out of the kidney by body wall movement, particularly in large or obese patients.

The skin suture should provide:

- Drainage around the nephrostomy tube as well as through it, i.e.: the nephrostomy acts as a conventional drain tube as well as an internal draining conduit.
- Comfort for the patient
- Stability of the loop within the kidney so that it remains tension free, even with body wall movement and respiration.

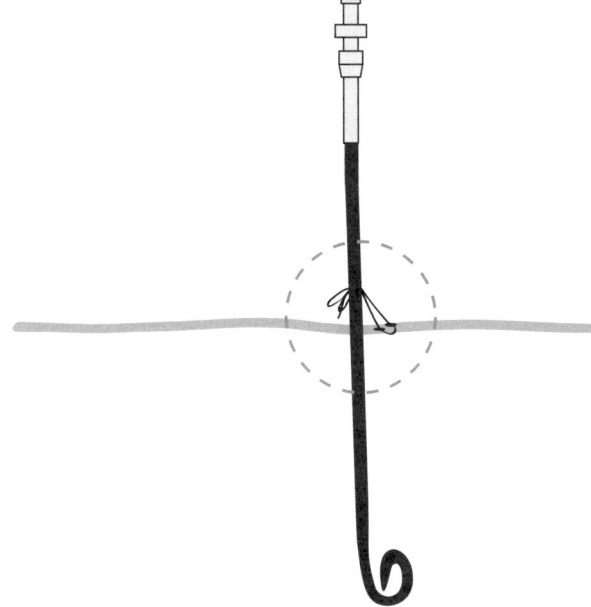

Fig. 5.13 The "mesentry" skin suture fixing the Cope nephrostomy to the skin but still allowing differential movement of the tube and body wall

Technique of Cope Nephrostomy Suture

A 2/0 silk on a cutting edge needle is passed through one edge of the nephrostomy incision, so the nephrostomy incision is not closed and hence can drain naturally around, as well as through the tube.

The suture is knotted on the skin edge, with equal lengths of suture remaining. A second knot is tied between the suture ends 1½ cm from the skin. This becomes the suture "mesentery".

The free ends of the suture are then tied firmly to the shaft of the "Cope" nephrostomy, again 1½ cm outside the skin.

This allows the "Cope" tubing to move in and out with breathing or body wall movement without tension developing between the skin and the kidney.

A coloplast nephrostomy bag is applied to the skin over the nephrostomy site.

Post-operative Care of the Nephrostomy

The Nephrostomy should be left on free drainage. I do not routinely spigot the nephrostomy. I will occasionally spigot the nephrostomy for situations such as PCNL in a solitary kidney, or when small stone fragments are seen in the distal ureter in the post PCNL KUB. A plain KUB should be performed after 24 h to assess the stone free status.

The nephrostomy can usually be removed 24–48 h post-surgery, providing the imaging demonstrates no residual calculi, and the patient is mobile and well.

Nephrostogram

I do not routinely perform a nephrostogram following PCNL. However, if there is suspicion of a collecting system perforation, fragments are seen down the ureter or following PCNL in a solitary kidney, I will perform an antegrade nephrostogram.

If contrast flows freely into the bladder, and the patient is pain free and afebrile, the nephrostomy may be removed.

I do order a CT-Nephrostogram after a complex PCNL, to obtain an accurate record of the collecting system for subsequent PCNL, which is often the case in patients with neurogenic bladder or urinary diversions.

Chapter 6
Complex PCNL and Antegrade Endopyelotomy

Conventional PCNL is now essentially restricted to the management of complicated calculi. Routine stones can be managed simply by ESWL, FURS or "Mini Perc".

Therefore, the current indications for PCNL are essentially "those calculi that cannot be easily and safely managed by less invasive techniques". These include the following:

Complex Calculi

1. Large, partial or complete staghorn calculi, particularly those complicated by infection.
2. Large dense calculi that are too large or hard for ESWL, too large for FURS, or refractory to ESWL, e.g. cystine

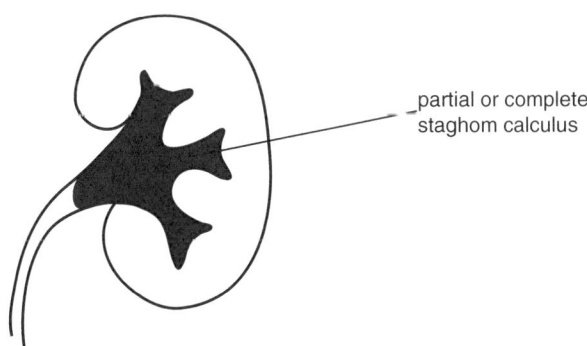

Fig. 6.1 Staghorn calculus

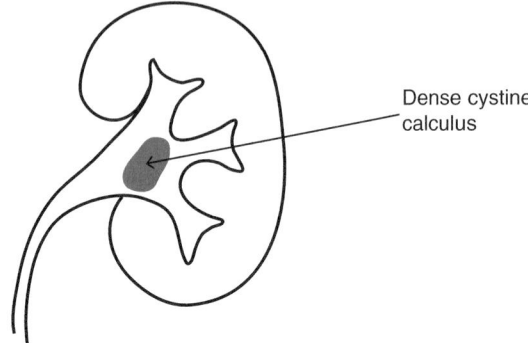

Fig. 6.2 Dense or hard calculi that do not fragment with ESWL

Complex Anatomy

1. Calculi associated with poor drainage, such as calculi in calyceal diverticulae, poorly draining lower pole calyces, pelviureteric junction obstructions or large impacted upper ureteric calculi.
2. Calculi associated with difficult access from the flank or the ureter, where the skin to kidney distance is too long for ESWL to focus and stones unsuitable for FURS, e.g. obesity, horseshoe kidney
3. Access requiring a supracostal track, e.g.:

    – Spina bifida associated with skeletal deformities
    – Calyceal diverticulum in the upper pole of the kidney
    – Staghorn calculus requiring upper pole access

4. Urinary diversions
5. Hydronephrosis with associated distended kidney and thin parenchyma

Fig. 6.3 Obstructing calculi associated with poor renal drainage

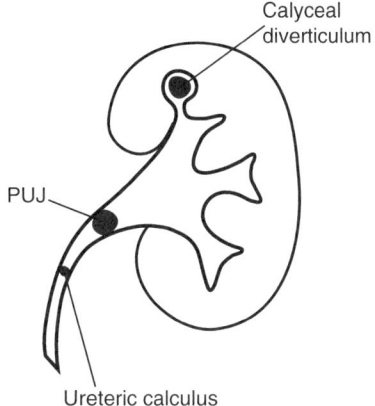

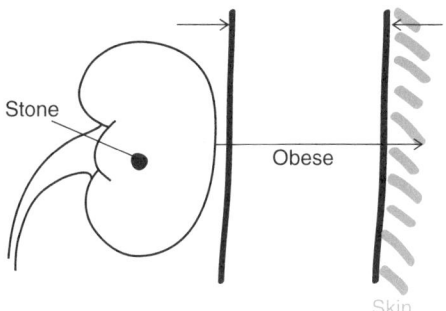

Fig. 6.4 An obese patient where the distance from the skin to the calculus exceeds the ESWL focal distance

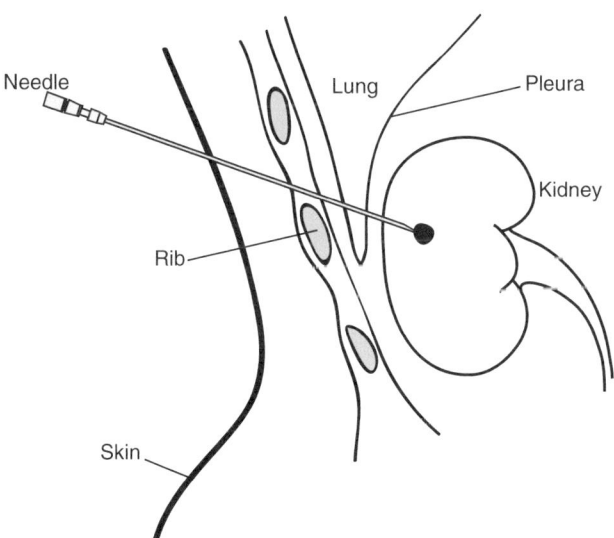

Fig. 6.5 A supracostal puncture track showing the surrounding structures

Fig. 6.6 Calculi in urinary diversions such as an ileal conduit

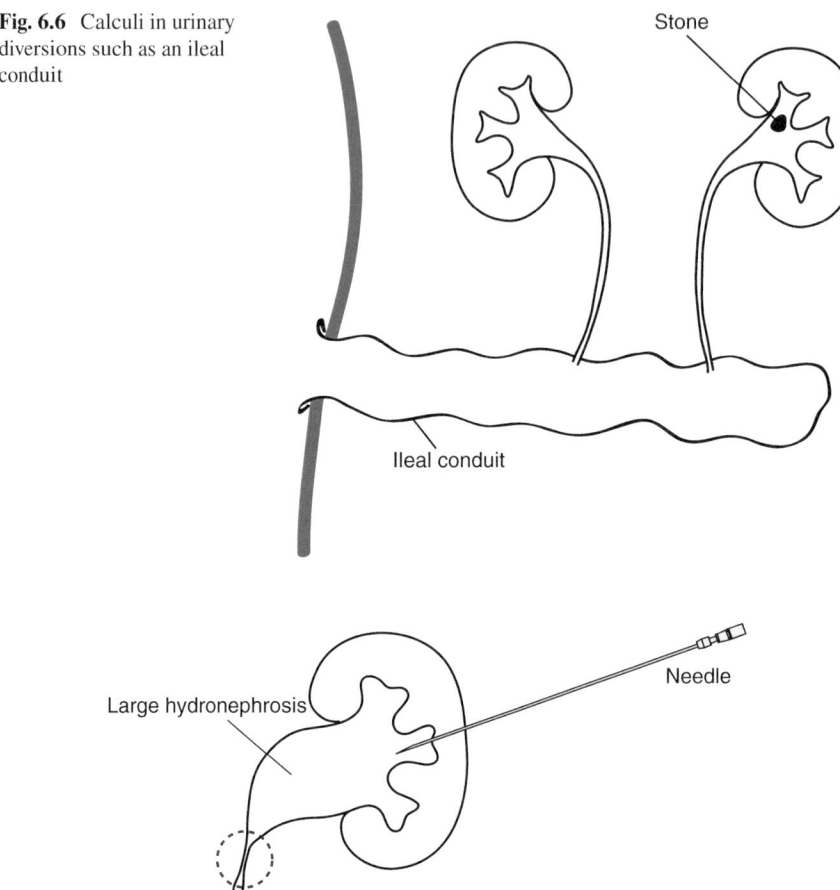

Fig. 6.7 A puncture into a hydronephrosis for antegrade endopyelotomy

Introduction

Until a surgeon has mastered the skills of basic PCNL, he or she should not attempt a difficult PCNL. Prior to surgery, the surgeon must evaluate the anatomy, develop an approach for primary and secondary punctures and anticipate difficulties and complications, both intra- and post-operatively

Specialised equipment must be sourced before commencing of the procedure, e.g. long PCNL sheath, long nephroscope, flexible nephroscope, holmium laser for horseshoe kidney, urethrotome with back cutting sickle knife for endopyelotomy, etc.

Advanced Skills Required for Difficult PCNL

- The surgeon must have mastered the techniques of accessing the kidney where there is little or no space to establish a guide wire in the collecting system.
- The surgeon must be familiar with the techniques and complications of supracostal puncture.
- The surgeon must be able to perform advanced punctures, e.g.
  - "Y" puncture
  - Target puncture
- Puncture of a large hydronephrosis.
- Obtaining renal access by utilising a guide wire in the retroperitoneum for the initial puncture.
- The techniques of antegrade ureteroscopy.
- Methylene blue and saline infusion to identify the direction of the renal pelvis.
- Creation of a "long Amplatz sheath".

These skills will be described in this chapter as they relate to specific clinical scenarios.

Scenario One: Large Infection-related Staghorn Calculus

Aim

Complete clearance of all infection-related stone by primary PCNL or combined therapy.

Potential Problems

- Incomplete clearance due to the length of the procedure, renal and stone anatomy or difficult percutaneous access
- Pyonephrosis, septicaemia or septic shock
- Difficult access, particularly when the calculus fills the collecting system with minimal space between the calculus and the collecting system in which to establish a stable guide wire

Preoperative Tests, Treatment and Precautions

- Patients must have a urine culture and (even if urine is sterile), parenteral antibiotics 48 h prior to procedure.
- Cross match two units of blood.

CT-IVP

Assessment of the stone:

- In a large stone, with a centrally placed stone mass and wide short calyces that can be easily accessed by two to three tracks, the surgeon should plan for complete primary clearance by PCNL.
- Assessment of the Hounsfield Unit (HU) of the calculus can help with preparation.
- An opaque or faintly opaque stone with a HU less than 400 is more likely to be struvite, hence softer and amenable to fragmentation by sonotrode. Conversely, higher HUs, above 500 and particularly towards or above 1000, tend to be calcium oxalate or calcium monohydrate, dense hard calculi that will almost certainly require ballistic lithotripsy.

The aim of surgery in this scenario is to completely clear the pelvic stone and as much of the peripheral stone volume as possible.

The peripheral calculi usually require two or even three separate "Target" or "Y" punctures for clearance.

The surgeon should commence by creating a primary track that will give access for removal of the majority of the stone bulk, including the central stone mass. If it is anticipated that the procedure may not be completed in one session, subsequent punctures should target those calyces with the poorest drainage. Further management of residual calculi will then be ESWL, PCNL, FURS or observation.

Scenario One: Large Infection-related Staghorn Calculus

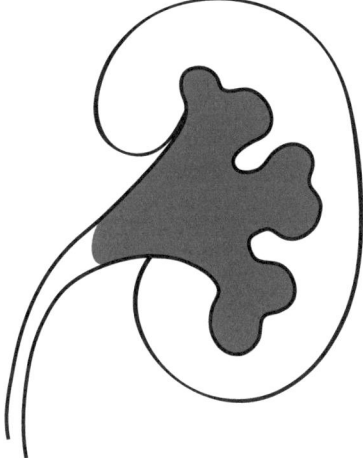

Fig. 6.8 A struvite staghorn calculus with a large central stone mass and short, wide calyceal extensions suitable for complete clearance by PCNL monotherapy

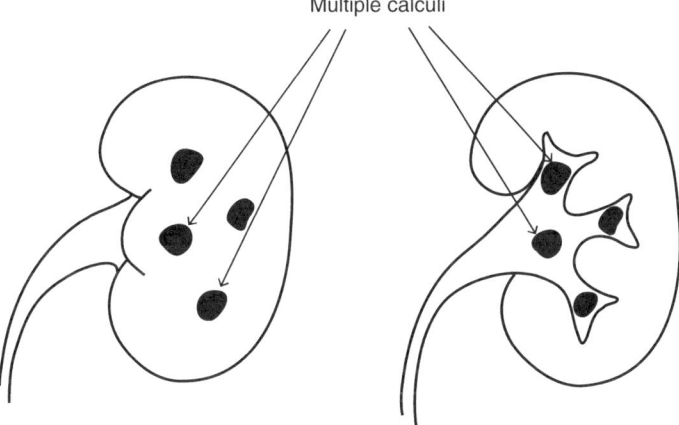

Fig. 6.9 Multiple peripheral calculi without a large central stone mass that may require an initial PCNL and subsequent PCNL, FURS or ESWL for complete clearance

Pyonephrosis

If the initial PCNL puncture aspirates frank pus, a nephrostomy should be inserted and the PCNL abandoned. The PCNL can be safely re-attempted following 5–7 days of percutaneous drainage and parental antibiotics. Failure to observe this precaution can result in the rapid development of septic shock.

Difficulties Encountered with Punctures for Complete Staghorn Calculi

It is usually easy to place the tip of the needle on the outer edge of a staghorn calculus, as the stone is big, easy to see on imaging, and can be felt when the needle tip contacts the stone. However, it is often difficult or impossible to thread a guide wire into the collecting system between the stone and the calyceal wall.

The surgeon has to establish a stable guide wire before being able to dilate a track onto the stone. This situation commonly arises when the needle hits the outer edge of the calyceal calculus. Little or no contrast can be aspirated and it is not possible to pass the tip of the guide wire between the stone and the collecting system.

This suggests that the needle is hitting the stone "end on". The surgeon must make a new puncture, with the aim of placing the needle tip just proximal to the outer end parallel to and along the side of the neck of the calyceal extension of the calculus. The intention is for the needle to slide between the stone and the collecting system. Occasionally, gentle "over distension" by retrograde injection of contrast or saline through the RGC may separate and create some space between the stone and the calyceal wall. However, one must exercise caution to avoid contrast extravasation and sepsis from forcing infected urine into the renal tissue.

If this is successful and the wire passes between the stone and the collecting system, a track can be dilated onto the tip of the stone, which is then excavated with the sonotrode.

If one cannot advance sufficient guide wire to obtain a stable track, the straight wire should be removed and exchanged for a J wire.

As the J wire is advanced, its rounded leading edge will often "roll" between the stone and calyceal wall to create a space sufficient to introduce enough guide wire into the kidney for dilatation of the track.

In the event of the above procedures failing to establish a stable length of guide wire within the collecting system for dilatation, the "retroperitoneal guide wire" (RPGW) technique can be employed.

After all attempts to introduce a guide wire into the collecting system have failed, re-puncture and advance the nephrostomy needle to touch the outer edge of the calyceal extension of the calculus.

Gently angle the needle and continue to pass it through the renal substance until it exits into the retroperitoneum. Having felt the stone by crepitus with the puncture, the needle and subsequently the guide wire will be in direct contact with the calculus.

After the needle has been advanced into the retroperitoneum, the needle and stylet are removed, leaving only the sheath in situ. A floppy-tipped hydrophilic guide wire is then introduced into the needle sheath and advanced so that it passes the stone and coils in the retroperitoneum.

This coiling gives the wire stability and allows the surgeon to dilate directly onto the stone.

By using one of the above techniques, the surgeon has established a stable guide wire for track dilatation. Now there is a guide wire adjacent to the calculus, the surgeon can make a track to the outer edge of the kidney. However, there will still be insufficient space between the stone and the collecting system to allow safe insertion of an Amplatz sheath or the nephroscope. A nephrotomy must now be developed so that the surgeon can see the calculus and create a cavity sufficient for the Amplatz sheath to safely enter the kidney.

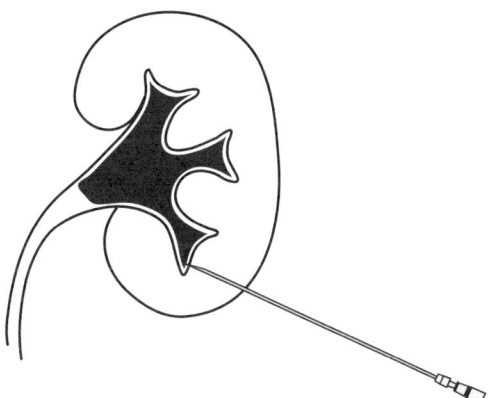

Fig. 6.10 The PCN needle contacting the outer edge of the calyceal extension

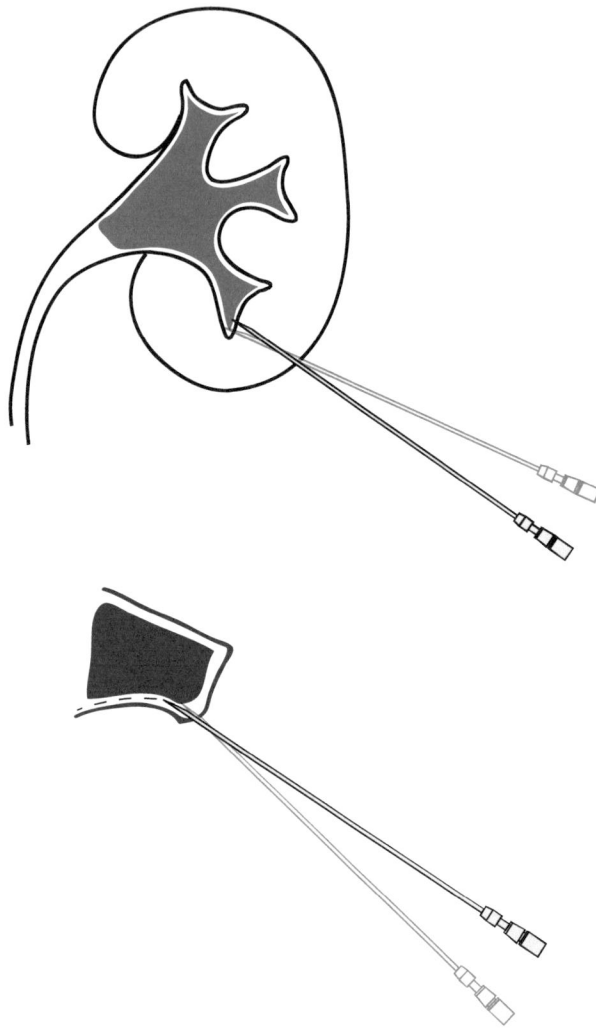

Fig. 6.11 The diagram above shows the needle hitting the outer border of the calculus end at 90°. The lower diagram demonstrates the re-puncture, onto the distal neck of the calyceal extension, parallel to and between the calyceal wall and the stone

Scenario One: Large Infection-related Staghorn Calculus

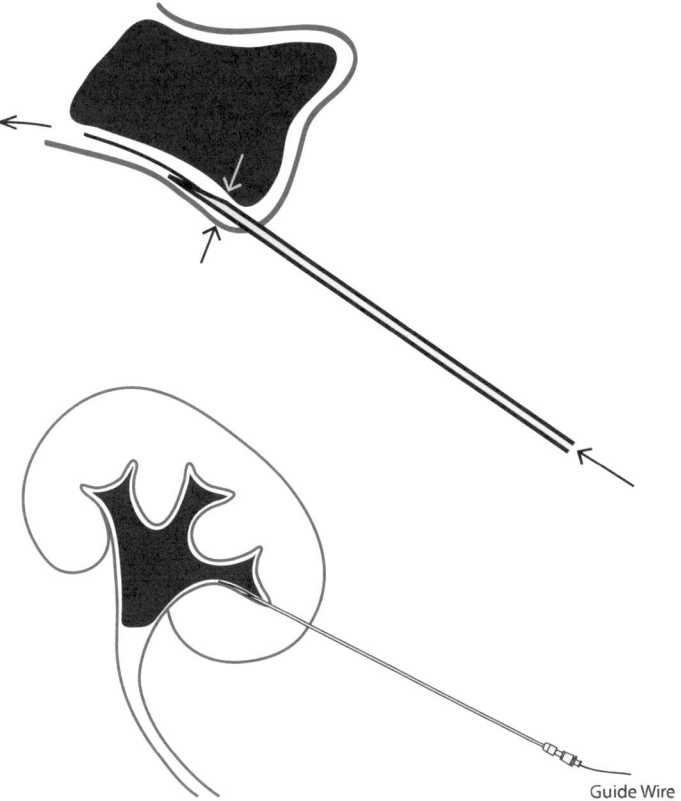

Fig. 6.12 The *upper diagram* demonstrates the puncture into the gap between the stone and calyx, allowing the guide wire to be advanced medially (*lower diagram*)

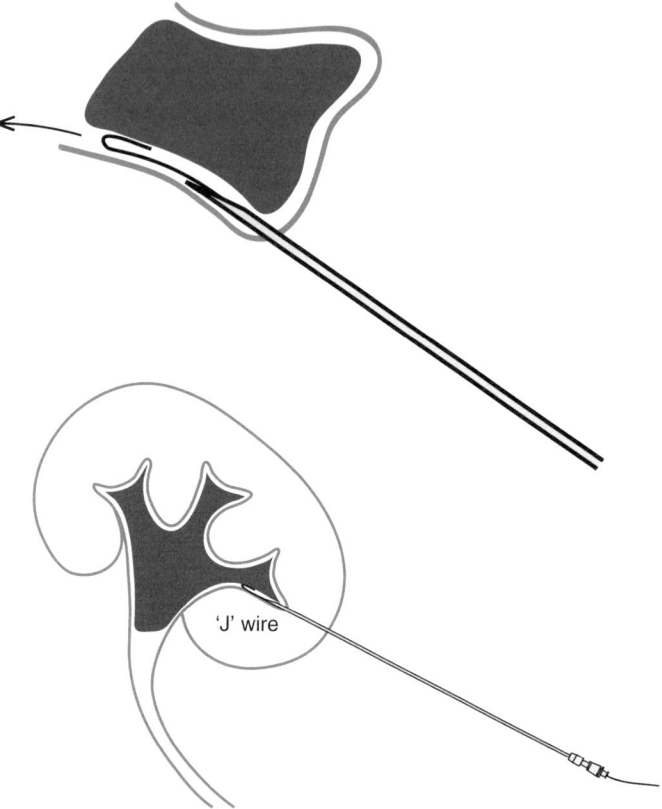

Fig. 6.13 Although the puncture has accessed the space between the stone and collecting system, the straight wire will not advance. By exchanging the straight wire with a "J wire", the "rolling edge" will often work its way along between the stone and the calyceal wall

Scenario One: Large Infection-related Staghorn Calculus

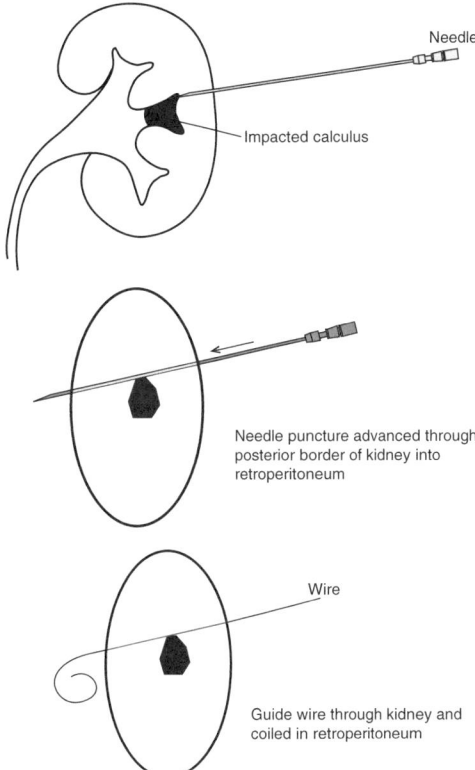

Fig. 6.14 The first stage of the RPGW technique. The stone is located by crepitus on contact with the needle. The needle is advanced through the kidney and a floppy-tipped guide wire threaded into the retroperitoneum until it is seen to coil

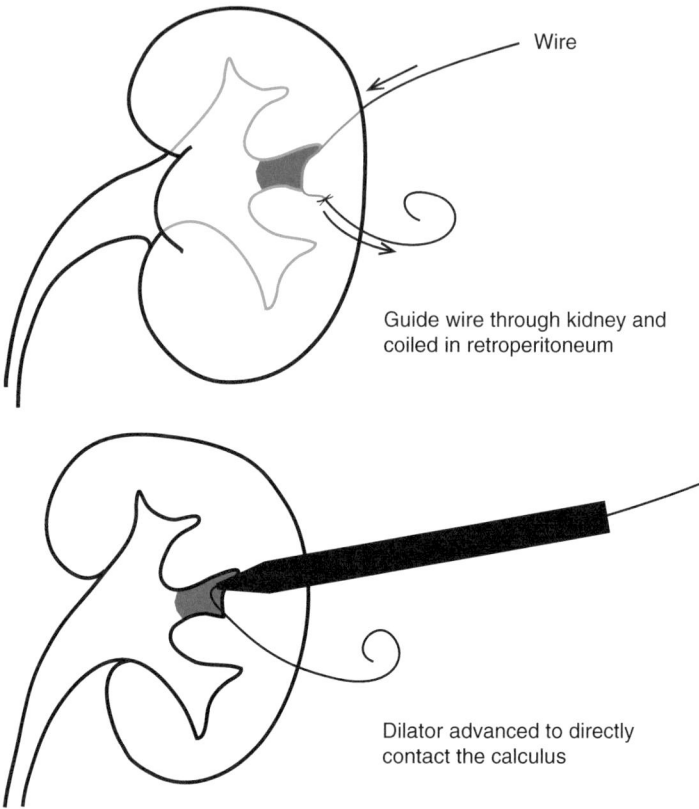

Fig. 6.15 Second-stage RPGW technique. The dilator is advanced until the tip contacts the stone. This can be confirmed by screening, "reverse parallax" and crepitus

Technique of Creating an Endoscopic Nephrotomy

Following the establishment of a guide wire adjacent to the stone using one of the above techniques, a 26 Fr dilator (I use a single stage) is advanced under II monitoring over the guide wire until the tip of the dilator is touching the calculus.

This is determined by screening, Parallax and the sensation of crepitus when the dilator tip contacts the stone.

The dilator should not be advanced further. Forcing the dilator between the calculus and the kidney will split the parenchyma and cause bleeding.

An Amplatz sheath is passed over the dilator until its leading edge is flush with the shoulder of the dilator. This is confirmed on II and the proximal dilator shaft marker if using the Webb dilator If the dilator is barely in the kidney, reverse the Amplatz sheath so the flat or non oblique end abuts the renal capsule.

An experienced assistant is required because they must maintain the Amplatz sheath precisely after removal of the dilator. A nephroscope is passed through the Amplatz sheath alongside the guide wire.

All clots within the Amplatz sheath are removed using alligator forceps.

The blunt tips of the alligator forceps are gently inserted alongside the guide wire through the parenchyma and opened, to separate the parenchyma, similar to creating an open nephrotomy. This is continued until the stone is visible.

When the stone is visible, it is safe to gently advance the nephroscope (but not the Amplatz sheath), to excavate a sufficient volume of stone using a sonotrode to create a cavity large enough for the safe advancement of the Amplatz sheath, either under direct vision or by reintroducing the dilator into the calyx.

At this stage, it is helpful to establish a guide wire into the collecting system. This will stabilise the track and enable the surgeon to introduce larger dilators and Amplatz sheaths for more efficient removal of the calculus.

By the time the surgeon has excavated enough stone for the Amplatz sheath to enter the calyx, it is usually possible to thread a second guide wire under vision between the calyceal wall and the stone, parallel to both of them, until the wire enters the renal pelvis and if fortunate, goes down the ureter.

A useful aid for determining the direction of the renal pelvis is the retrograde infusion of methylene blue solution.

A pre-prepared solution of normal saline and methylene blue is infused through the retrograde catheter by the assistant.

The surgeon is directed by the blue flushes to the space between the stone and calyceal wall, which indicates the direction in which to pass the guide wire through the nephroscope, or further excavate with the sonotrode. As the stone bulk is reduced, the methylene blue infusion becomes more profuse and the path for the guide wire clearer.

As soon as the surgeon reaches the renal pelvis, a UGW should be established.

Before introducing the UGW from the bladder end of the RGC, the assistant must remove the minimum volume extension tubing from the Leur lock. The assistant then introduces the floppy end of a straight hydrophilic guide wire into the ureteric catheter and threads it towards the kidney.

The surgeon identifies the wire endoscopically as it enters the pelvis.

It can be confusing as to whether the wire seen in the pelvis is the nephrostomy or the retrograde wire.

If the assistant "wiggles" the ureteric wire up and down, this manoeuvre identifies the UGW. If not, II screening will assist the surgeon in identifying the correct wire.

Once the UGW is identified, it is grasped by the surgeon and extracted through the Amplatz sheath. Both ends of the UGW are then grasped with artery forceps, which are separately fixed to the drapes at either end.

Now the PNCL becomes straightforward and safe as the guide wire cannot be displaced. It becomes now a simple procedure for the surgeon to upsize the nephrostomy track size to 28 or 32 Fr over the UGW. The larger sheath size greatly facilitates flushing, irrigation, vision and stone removal.

If the stone is hard and large, it is usually more efficient at this stage to exchange the ultrasonic lithotrite for the pneumatic lithoclast.

The PCNL should proceed through this primary track until all visible stone has been cleared.

Once this is achieved, the surgeon must assess the progress of the procedure.

It is generally accepted that even an uncomplicated PCNL should not continue in excess of 2 h of nephroscopy.

After this period, the incidence of blood loss, infection, patient instability and "TUR syndrome" increases significantly. It is always acceptable to place a small "Cope" nephrostomy and complete the PCNL safely at a later date.

Therefore, if more than 2 h has elapsed or the patient is unstable, a nephrostomy should be inserted and the procedure terminated.

If the stone along the primary track is cleared, the patient is stable, and less than 2 h have elapsed, the PCNL may continue, usually requiring two or more separate targeted nephrostomies.

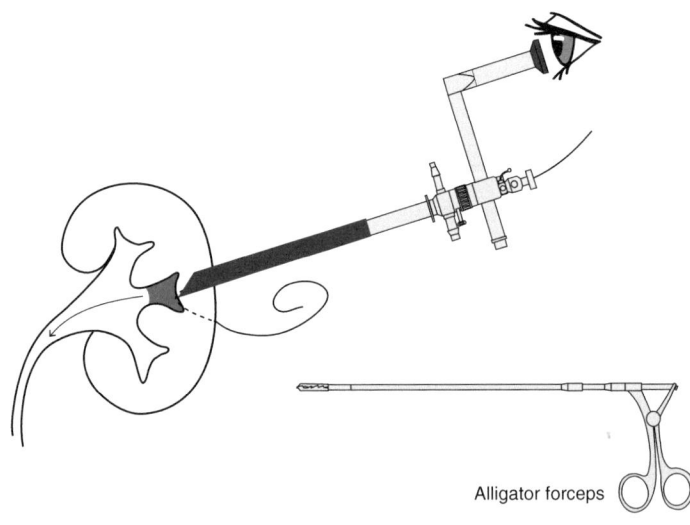

Fig. 6.16 The first stage of an endoscopic nephrotomy, the Amplatz sheath is advanced as close to the stone as possible over a dilator without splitting the parenchyma and the surgeon looks into the sheath following the guide wire

Scenario One: Large Infection-related Staghorn Calculus

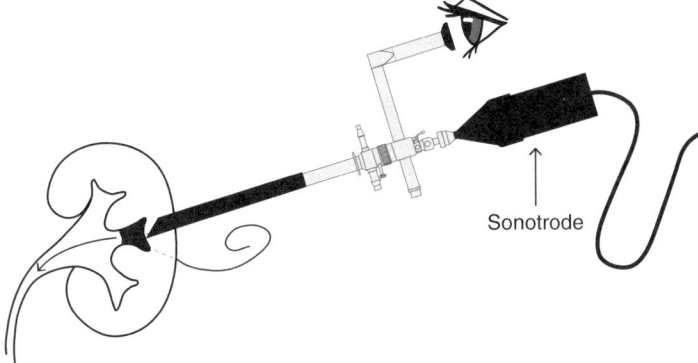

Fig. 6.17 Excavation of the outer stone in the calyx through the endoscopic nephrotomy to create a cavity for the introduction of the Amplatz sheath into the calyx

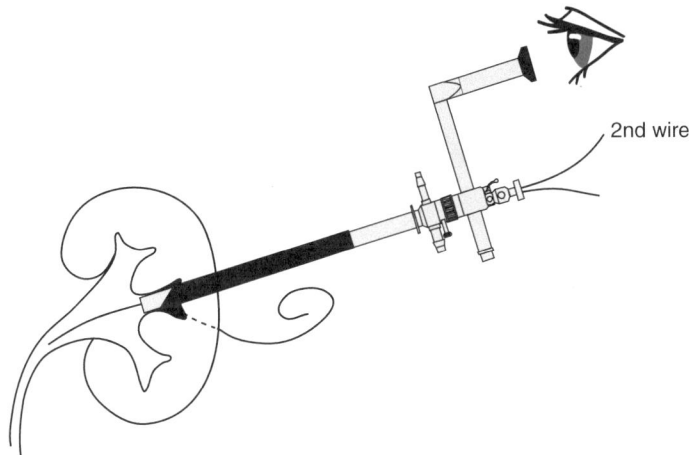

Fig. 6.18 Endoscopic placement of a guide wire into the collecting system after introduction of the Amplatz sheath. Often, although stone and the calyceal wall are visible, it is not clear which is the most direct route from the calyx to the renal pelvis

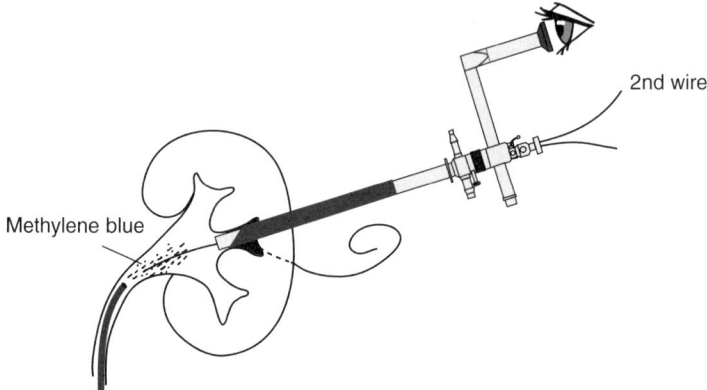

Fig. 6.19 Identification of the direction to the renal pelvis using RG injection of a saline and methylene blue solution

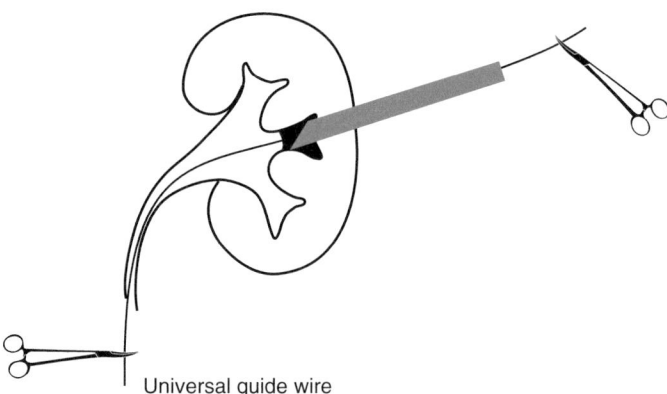

Fig. 6.20 Establishment of UGW

Supplementary Target Punctures during Staghorn Calculus Removal

The existing Amplatz sheath should be left in situ.

This tamponades the existing track and fixes the kidney, making further punctures easier. The sheath also acts as an excellent venting drain for blood, irrigant and stone fragments during PCNL through other calyces. Having punctured a secondary calyx, a modified "calyx to calyx UGW" can be established, which provides increased stability for the subsequent dilatations.

I usually find that the primary or initial track is the best site for the nephrostomy at the end of the PCNL. Before placing the final nephrostomy tube, the initial track should be reinspected. In most cases, copious stone and blood clot will be in the renal pelvis, having fallen centrally during clearing of the secondary stone extensions. This debris must be cleared before final imaging and nephrostomy insertion.

The needle track should be aligned parallel to the axis of the targeted calyx.

The surgeon will know the needle is on the targeted stone by the sensation of crepitus. Due to the existing Amplatz sheath draining the kidney, it is not usually possible to inject sufficient contrast into the targeted calyx to assist with the secondary target puncture.

Following the needle puncture, a straight floppy-tipped hydrophilic guide wire is threaded through the needle sheath, past the stone and into the renal pelvis.

The guide wire is extracted from the original nephrostomy, both ends are clamped, to create a modified UGW, from calyx to calyx.

The wire into the targeted calyx is now stable, and it is safe to dilate onto the stone. This secondary UGW is not essential, but if it can be created, it is very useful for the puncture and subsequent clearance of the stone fragments from the calyx and renal pelvis.

The original sheath provides excellent drainage and acts as a low pressure vent for stone fragments and clots, as the PCNL continues.

Once the targeted calyx is endoscopically clear, the renal pelvis should be re-endoscoped through the primary sheath. Considerable debris will usually have passed from the targeted calyx.

I find that after extensive ultrasonic or ballistic lithotripsy that there are often multiple scattered fine 2–3 mm stone fragments that are too numerous, small or hidden in clot, to extract manually. These can be cleared very effectively by a saline flush through single or multiple Amplatz sheaths. Attach a medium-sized infant feeding tube (IFT) to a 20 cc syringe of normal saline. Introduce the tip of the IFT deep to the sheath and flush gently. As the sheath is a wide and open system, stone fragments and clot readily flush out without increasing intrarenal pressure.

If the patient is stable and there is time, further similar punctures can be made. If not, a "Cope" loop nephrostomy is inserted via the original Amplatz sheath, and the secondary access sheaths removed. Nephrostomies are not necessary for the secondary punctures.

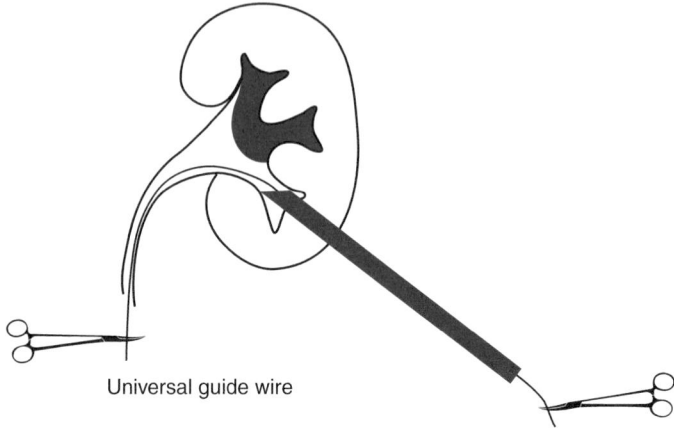

Fig. 6.21 Before performing secondary nephrostomies, a UGW is established to maintain the primary track and stabilise the kidney. Separate target punctures, in the presence of an Amplatz sheath, do not need to be larger than 26 Fr. If the stone extension is not large, the Mini-PCNL instruments are very useful for secondary punctures

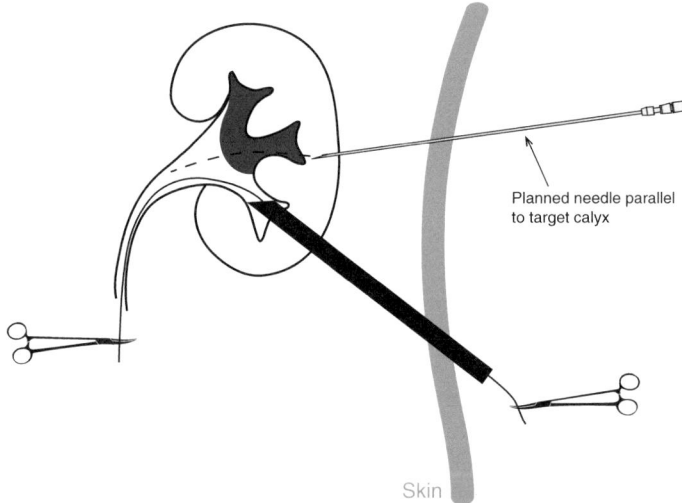

Fig. 6.22 Second calyceal puncture. The original Amplatz sheath is left to provide drainage and stabilise the kidney for the second puncture

Scenario One: Large Infection-related Staghorn Calculus

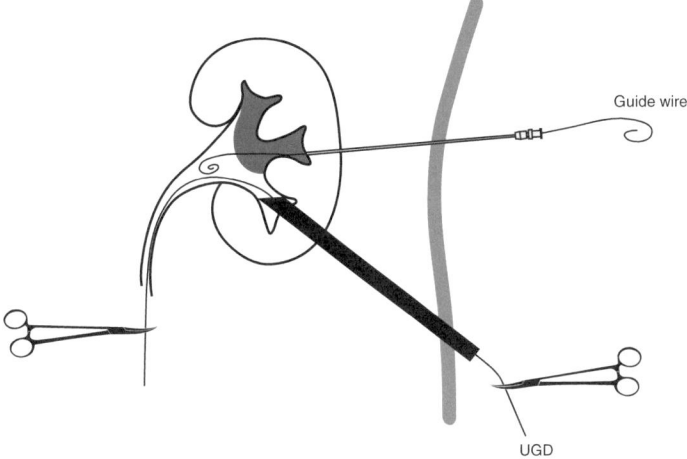

Fig. 6.23 Secondary calyx puncture and introduction of a guide wire into the renal pelvis

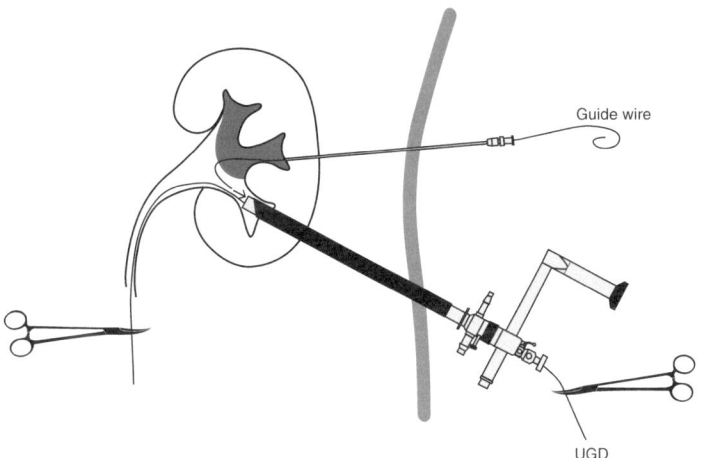

Fig. 6.24 The new guide wire is grasped by the surgeon through the original Amplatz sheath

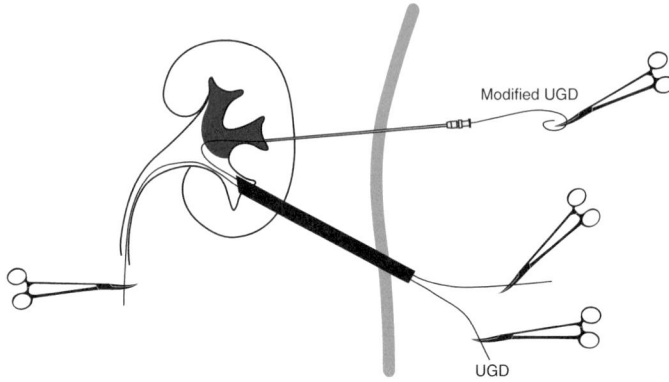

Fig. 6.25 Extraction and fixation of the second guide wire to establish a modified calyx to calyx secondary UGW

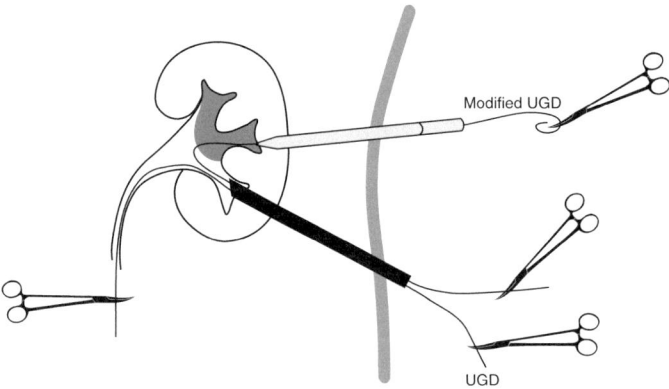

Fig. 6.26 Dilation is now straightforward over the stabilised modified UGW

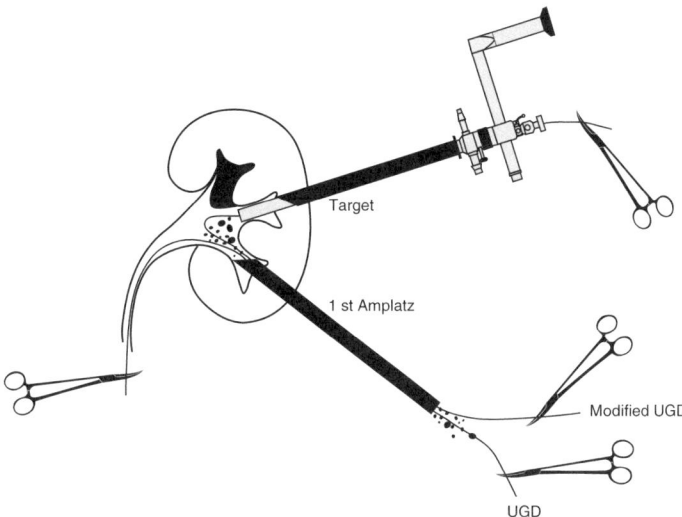

Fig. 6.27 During nephrolithotomy through the secondary track, stone fragments and irrigant freely exit from the primary Amplatz sheath

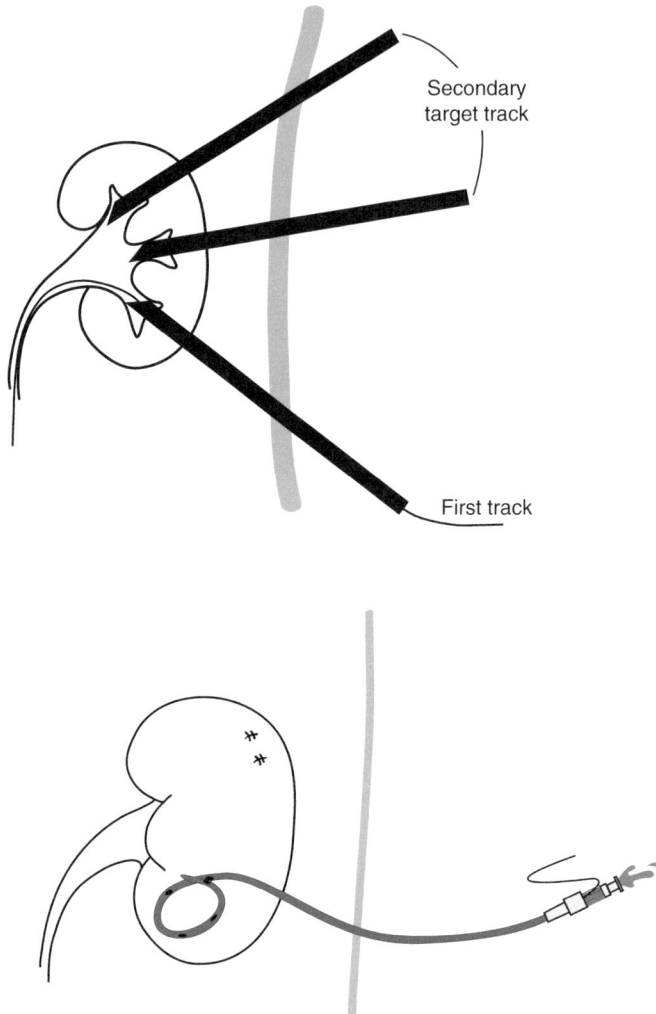

Fig. 6.28 Nephrostomy at the termination of a complex PCNL – only one nephrostomy is needed, the other tracks will close spontaneously

Scenario Two: Complex Recurrent Infection Calculi Associated with a Chronically Infected Urinary Diversion or Associated Neurogenic Bladder

Difficulties and problems anticipated:

1. Urine infection
   In spite of medical therapy and stone clearance, the infection is never cleared, due to the underlying anatomical abnormality of the urinary drainage.
2. Difficulties with access:
   - Paraplegia, spina bifida, kyphoscoliosis
   - Urinary diversion
     In most of these patients, it is often not possible to establish retrograde ureteric catheter access at the time of the PCNL due to the urinary diversion or neurogenic bladder.
3. Anaesthesia difficulties:
   - Hyperreflexia
4. Decubitus ulceration

Indications for Stone Removal

1. Obstruction
2. Sepsis
3. Decreased renal function

Aims of Treatment

Stone "palliation". In other words, to safely remove as much stone as possible, if not all, to relieve obstruction of the ureter, pelvis or calyces and to reduce stone volume, knowing that repeat procedures will almost certainly be required in the future, whatever the outcome of this PCNL.

Pre-admission

- CT-IVP to assess the following:
  - Kyphoscoliosis
  - Limb and body wall contractures
  - Anatomy of the stone, kidney and collecting system

- Renal malrotation
- Assess the relationships of the kidney and the possibility of supracostal approach
- Identify organs (e.g. bowel, lung pleura) adjacent to the kidney
- Plan the primary and possibly secondary nephrostomy approaches

Preoperative Preparation

- Admit 48 h prior to surgery for insertion of a radiological nephrostomy to:
  - Obtain urine for M C & S
  - Unobstruct kidneys
  - Avoid urosepsis
  - Provide a conduit for contrast infusion at the time of PCNL (as retrograde access may not be possible)

Other Preparation

- Commence parenteral antibiotics after the nephrostomy urine culture taken (even if urine culture is negative)
- Cross-match four units of blood
- Elective booking for post-operative ICU admission to monitor
  - Sepsis
  - Fluid volume
  - Temperature

Theatre: Additional Equipment

- Military "trauma bean bag" for safely maintaining the position and avoiding pressure points in patients with skeletal abnormalities during the PCNL
- Flexible cystoscope (may be required to endoscope a conduit or bladder if there are skeletal or urinary drainage abnormalities.)

Aims of Surgery

- If possible and safe, clear all calculi.
- If complete clearance is not possible, remove the major bulk of stone.
- Remove all calculi causing intrarenal or ureteric obstruction.

Ileal Conduit

When preparing and positioning the patient for surgery, ensure that the ileal conduit stoma is exposed.

Insert a Foley catheter into the conduit. It is often possible to infuse sufficient contrast through a Foley catheter in an ileal conduit to image the ureters and renal collecting system.

However, as good imaging cannot be guaranteed, I routinely arrange for the patient to have a preoperative radiological nephrostomy for contrast infusion.

Surgical Approach

As described earlier for a complex staghorn calculus.

Attempt to establish a guide wire into the conduit and a UGW through the conduit if possible (flexible cystoscope).

The extent and aims of the PCNL should be planned prior to surgery. The operative aim is to remove as much stone as safely as possible with a priority to removing all obstructing calculi.

Avoid overzealous and long procedures. These patients are more prone to urosepsis, bleeding, volume movement and decubitus ulceration.

Also, they will commonly develop new calculi, even after complete clearance.

Remember, the aim is pragmatic "stone palliation".

If complete stone clearance is safely achieved, this is a bonus.

Scenario Three: Calculi Within Calyceal Diverticulae

Anticipated Difficulties

Calyceal diverticulae (CD) are often polar. Therefore, the puncture is into the region of the kidney that is most mobile and prone to rotation and "flipping".

Access to an upper pole CD may require a supracostal or transpleural nephrostomy.

Calculi may completely fill the entire diverticular cavity, leaving no space for a guide wire to coil or contrast to delineate.

CD are often small targets.

When a CD is filled with multiple small stones, the calculi can be very difficult to "feel" by the sensation of crepitus with the puncture needle. These "calculi" often turn out to be very fine sand. Crepitus is a useful sign and aids in accessing a CD, as it may not be possible to outline the diverticulae with contrast, but the stones need to be solid to elicit crepitus. It is very useful to employ the technique of "reverse parallax" imaging when puncturing a CD because the absence of "crepitus feedback" when the contents are only fine sand can compromise the surgeon's confidence that the needle tip is inside the CD.

It is most uncommon to be able to pass a guide wire into a calyceal diverticulum and for the wire to spontaneously continue down the infundibular stalk into the calyx and pelvis because the stalks tend to be narrow and eccentric. The surgeon must be prepared for a difficult puncture.

Even if a small amount of wire can be coiled within the CD, it can still be easily displaced during track dilatation.

An upper pole CD may require a supracostal approach.

When a nephroscope is introduced into a calyceal diverticulum, it is easy to lose the track, because the cavity is small and guide wire stability is tenuous.

One must plan to clear the stone with as little excursion of the nephroscope as possible.

Aims of the Puncture for Treatment of Stones in a Calyceal Diverticulum

- To create a stable track for dilatation into the calyceal diverticulum
- To completely clear the calculi

I have not been convinced that attempts at endoscopic ablation or marsupialisation of the cavity are successful, enduring or necessary.

If calculi recur, the anatomical abnormality should be removed. This is a rare situation and best treated by laparoscopic or robotic partial nephrectomy. It is the anatomy of the CD that has caused the stone in the first place.

Preparation Prior to Surgery for Calculi in Calyceal Diverticulae

CT-IVU: Points to Observe

Stone

- It is critical to know exactly where the stone is in relation to the collecting system and the kidney, e.g. anterior and posterior.

Collecting system

- It is very important to know the size and disposition of the CD for the initial puncture, as well as the adjacent calyceal anatomy. It may be necessary to do an elective "Y puncture" when stable calyceal access cannot be achieved by the primary puncture.

Scenario Three: Calculi Within Calyceal Diverticulae

Methylene blue saline infusion (MBSI)

- Once the nephroscope is within the CD, MBSI can be very useful to locate the infundibular stalk. The stalk can then be cannulated directly by passing a guide wire through the nephroscope into the stalk along the calyx into the renal pelvis and ureter, creating a very stable track.

Potential Scenarios After Needle Puncture of a Calyceal Diverticulum

(a) After puncturing the diverticulum, the guide wire passes down the infundibulum into the associated calyx, and down the ureter. This is an extremely rare but most pleasing experience. In this scenario, dilatation can proceed directly over the guide wire.
(b) The guide wire enters the diverticulum and circles around the stone. This occurs in larger calyceal diverticula, and is usually sufficient for a successful dilatation into the diverticulum.
(c) The guide wire hits the stone but will not coil within the diverticulum or around the stone, nor will it enter the infundibular stalk. The options for this scenario are discussed below.

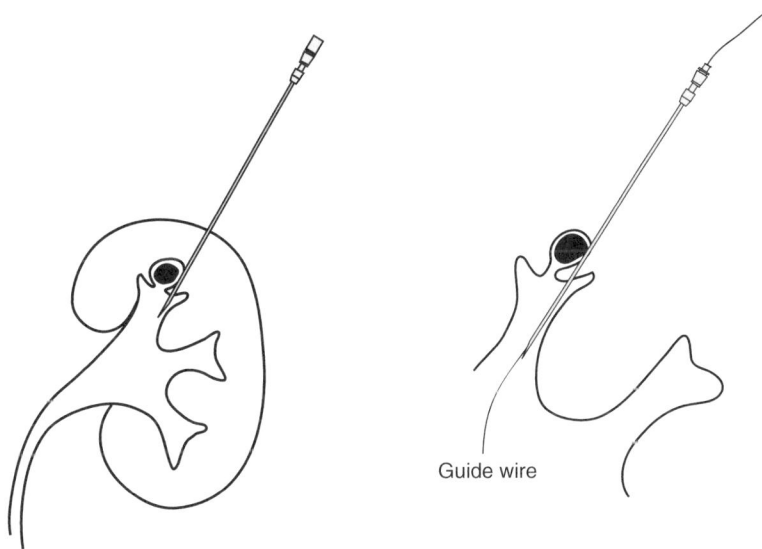

Fig. 6.29 If the stone can be "felt" but no wire can be introduced into the CD, the needle, which is in contact with the stone, can be advanced into the calyx related to the CD. Then a guide wire can be passed to the ureter and the subsequent dilation will be adjacent to and in direct contact with the calculus. This creates and provides endoscopic access for stone removal

Options

The needle, after touching the stone, can be advanced into the calyx directly (bypassing the CD stalk).

The guide wire can then be fed into the pelvis and down the ureter and dilatation performed onto the stone.

If this procedure fails, perform a "Y" puncture

- The "Y" puncture was originally devised for the management of the "parallel lie" stone.
- The "parallel lie" was a common scenario before three-dimensional CT imaging. A calyceal stone, which appeared to be in the line of the puncture on II screening, could not be located endoscopically, as it was lying in an anterior or posterior calyx, which was adjacent to, but parallel to the initial puncture. On II, it appeared that the puncture needle was in the calyx containing the calculus.

(a) As corresponding calyces are essentially parallel, it is impossible for a rigid or flexible endoscope to enter an adjacent calyx.
(b) As the calyces are close together, it is safe and simple to puncture the adjacent calyx, utilising the same body wall and outer parenchymal puncture entry site.

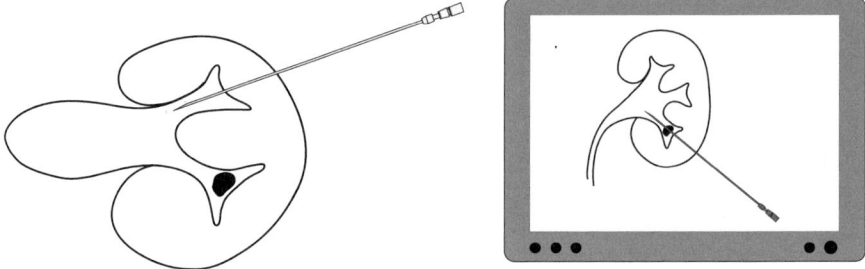

Fig. 6.30 The appearance of a "Parallel lie" on the monitor suggests on the vertical view that the needle is in the calyx containing the calculus

"Y" Puncture Technique

1. Pass a guide wire through the original puncture into the renal pelvis and down the ureter. This establishes the body wall track for the long arm of the "Y puncture", assists in stabilising the kidney and allows re-entry into the kidney if the "Y" puncture fails.
2. After endoscoping the initial calyx and passing a guide wire down the ureter, remove the Amplatz sheath.
3. Pass a PCNL puncture needle along the body wall component of the track under II screening.
4. Advance the needle until the tip of the needle contacts the stone in the adjacent calyx. This is confirmed by crepitus between the puncture needle and the stone, observing the stone being deflected by the needle during II screening and by "reverse parallax".
5. Remove the needle and stylet, pass a second guide wire alongside the calculus to enter the adjacent calyx, and thread the wire into the pelvis and ureter.
6. Re-introduce the dilator over this second guide wire, using the existing body wall track (the shaft of the "Y") and dilate directly onto the calculus. Insert an Amplatz sheath and remove the stone.

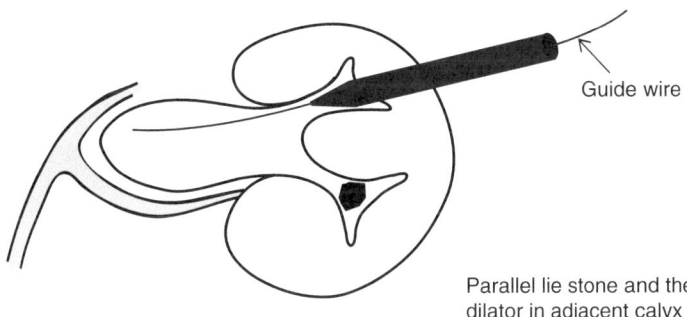

Fig. 6.31 "Y" puncture. First, establish a stable (or UGW) wire down the ureter. The kidney is now ready for the "Y" puncture

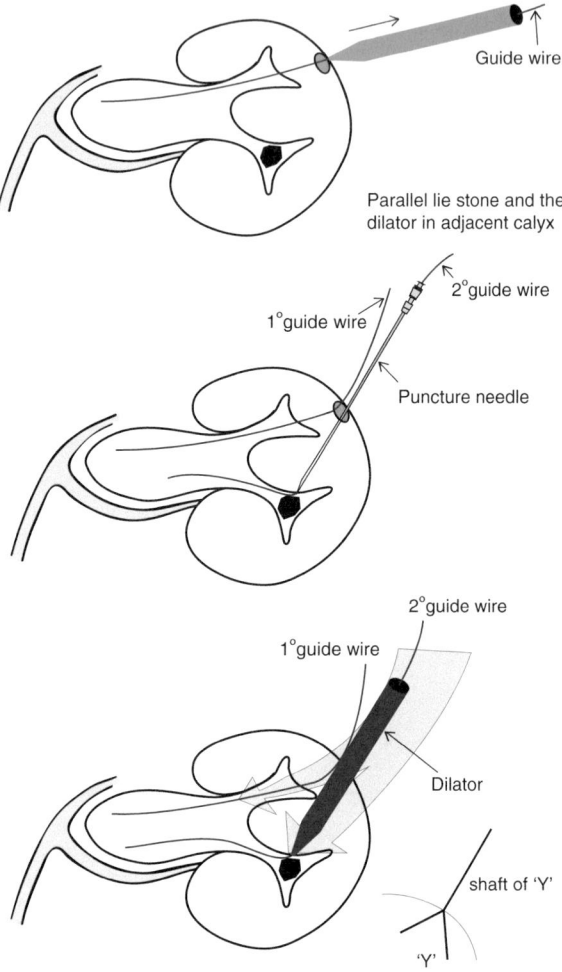

Fig. 6.32 The technique of the "Y" puncture

Application of the "Y" Puncture for Access into a Calyceal Diverticulum

When it is not possible to maintain a guide wire in the CD, remove the needle, and re-puncture the closest calyx to the diverticulum (previously identified on CT/IVU).

Pass a guide wire down the ureter to stabilise the track and the kidney.

Remove the Amplatz sheath, and perform a "Y puncture" onto the stone (as described above). The stone is identified by "crepitus" on the tip of the needle with confirmation by "reverse parallax".

Attempt to reintroduce the guide wire into the diverticulum, although this may not always be possible. If you cannot establish a stable wire within the diverticulum, pass the needle alongside the stone as previously described for the management of a complex staghorn calculus (see Fig. 6.15), so that the needle goes through the kidney and into the retroperitoneum (RPGW). Then introduce a new guide wire through the needle sheath after removing the needle and stylet.

The wire will lie adjacent to and in contact with the stone. The original guide wire in the adjacent calyx will stabilise the track. Using the same body wall track, pass a single-stage dilator directly onto the stone and enter the cavity with the sonotrode ready to aspirate the stone particles through this second limb of the "Y" puncture.

Complete the procedure by inserting a "Cope" nephrostomy through the original calyceal puncture.

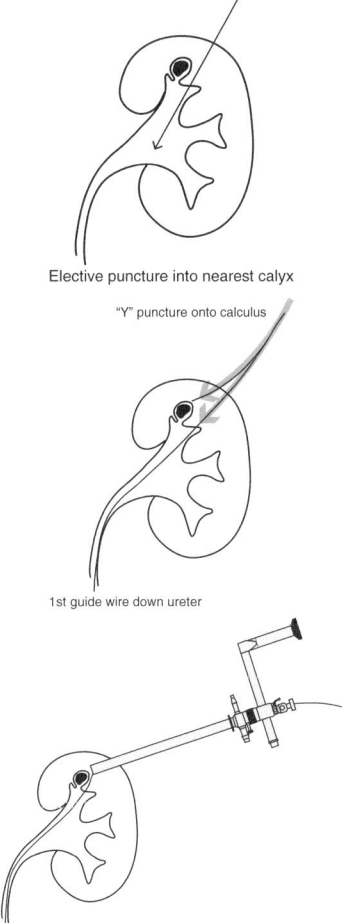

Fig. 6.33 "Y" puncture for CD

If the Guide Wire Will Not Enter the Diverticulum and There Is No Adjacent Calyx

In this scenario, puncture the kidney (as described in the Fig. 6.15) so that the needle tip directly contacts and passes the stone. Establish a retroperitoneal guide wire. Using a target dilator, dilate directly onto the stone and remove it. I find the ultrasonic aspirator ideal in this scenario.

As you have not entered the major collecting system with this approach, it may not be possible to leave a nephrostomy, which is not an issue. If you are concerned about extravasation or bleeding, a Yeates or Penrose drain tube can be pushed along the nephrostomy track with a finger to the edge of the kidney and sutured to the skin (as one would do after open surgery), unless the pleura has been transgressed. If that is the case, I do not leave a drain tube that would exit through the pleura.

Stone Removal from a Calyceal Diverticulum

No matter how well the track seems, both the track and the diverticulum can be easily lost during PCNL in a CD.

Therefore, the surgeon must avoid all unnecessary movements of the nephroscope and the Amplatz sheath.

It is critical to have an experienced assistant to maintain the guide wire and sheath.

The surgeon needs to be totally focused on the stone.

CD calculi can be very small and are often multiple, even though they look large and single on CT.

The surgeon should enter the CD with the sonotrode "at the ready". Aim to clear the entire stone mass before removing the nephroscope. Re-entry can be difficult, especially when the track is polar and unstable.

Drainage

Once the calculus is cleared, it may be possible to see the infundibulum stalk, but if not, have the assistant infuse saline and a methylene blue through the retrograde catheter.

Identify the infundibulum, pass a guide wire into the calyx and pelvis, and introduce a cope nephrostomy tube.

Scenario Three: Calculi Within Calyceal Diverticulae

If a "Y" puncture has been performed, insert the "Cope" nephrostomy into the adjacent calyx.

If the procedure has been routine without significant trauma, no nephrostomy is required.

A Yeates drain, Penrose tube or Cope nephrostomy can be placed alongside the kidney if extravasation or bleeding has occurred and one cannot insert a formal nephrostomy.

Alternatively, if the track is lost (not uncommon) and the procedure uncomplicated, no nephrostomy or external drain tube is required.

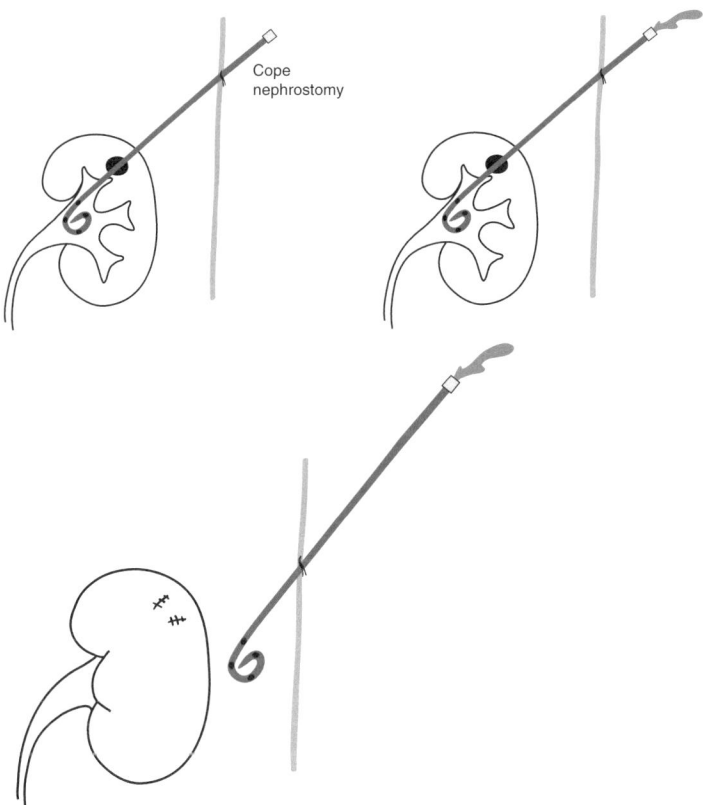

Fig. 6.34 On completion of PCNL in a CD, a Cope nephrostomy can be introduced through the infundibular stalk, the neighbouring calyx, or placed next to the kidney to function as a conventional drain tube

Scenario Four: The Management of Calculi in a Narrow or Poorly Draining Calyx, or a Stone Forming a Complete Cast of a Calyx

These are usually lower pole. Management is the same as for the removal of calculi in a calyceal diverticulum.

Scenario Five

Previous Renal Surgery

With a history of previous open renal surgery (usually a nephrolithotomy or extended pyelolithotomy), and particularly in patients with a past history of cystinuria, scarring of the perinephric region and the kidney will compromise a PCNL. Because of body wall and perirenal scarring and renal tissue rigidity, the kidney and collecting system are scarred and fixed. As a result, the parenchyma easily splits with dilation, intrarenal manipulation, and instrumentation.

Body wall scarring can be overcome using dilators or artery forceps and occasionally a blade, but access can still be difficult.

The surgeon loses tactile feedback with respect to depth of the dilator and level of the renal capsule. Because the track is rigid and firm, it often requires considerable force to dilate.

Increasing force on the dilator makes it more prone to suddenly "give", or jerk, which may result in a potentially uncontrolled forward lunge of the dilator and trauma to the kidney. The body wall component of the track can be dilated with artery forceps. The surgeon must be very cautious using this manoeuvre and not dilate too deeply, as the definition of normal anatomical planes is lost in scar and it is possible for the tips of the forceps to enter the kidney if strict radiological monitoring is not employed.

Using any form of dilation in a previously operated kidney can cause the kidney to split. I find that previously operated kidneys bleed more and tamponade less effectively than unoperated kidneys. I have a very low threshold for terminating PCNL and proceed to radiological embolisation for bleeding in patients with a history of previous surgery.

All forms of dilatation should be closely monitored by II.

In the presence of significant body wall scarring, it is my experience that Amplatz and SSD dilators have less friction and more flexibility and are easier to introduce than the telescoping metal or inflatable balloon dilators.

Whatever type of dilator system is employed, the surgeon must take precautions to avoid jerky and sudden advances of the dilator. This is done by firmly applying the ulnar surface of the dilating hand to the patient's back, preventing uncontrolled dilator advancement when scar tissue suddenly splits (see Fig. 5.4).

Renal Scarring

Due to fixation and tissue rigidity, scarred renal parenchyma is more solid and less "spongy" and therefore more prone to splitting. Splitting can extend into the collecting system and renal sinus.

This lack of suppleness often leads to significant bleeding. If the split extends into the renal sinus, it may damage segmental vessels. Tissue rigidity also decreases the mobility of the nephroscope. Even minor manipulation of the nephroscope in a scarred kidney can cause splitting and bleeding.

In patients with a history of previous percutaneous nephrolithotomies or open surgery, increased bleeding should be anticipated. Two units of blood should be cross-matched prior to PCNL and the patient warned of the increased possibility of transfusion and embolisation.

If significant bleeding is encountered early in a PCNL in the presence of renal scarring, it is prudent to cease the operation early, insert a nephrostomy and perform a repeat PCNL through a separate track a few weeks later.

Summary of the Management of Patient Undergoing PCNL in the Presence of Significant Renal and Perirenal Scarring

- Anticipate difficulties with bleeding and access:
- Cross-match two units of blood prior to surgery.
- If significant bleeding, cease the procedure early.
- If bleeding continues, refer for radiological embolisation early. These kidneys tend to bleed more than unoperated kidneys, as the parenchyma is more rigid and does not tamponade as well.
- Anticipate that the PCNL may need to be truncated. Have a priority plan to remove the most significant and obstructing calculi first.
- Discuss the potential outcome of incomplete stone clearance with the patient at the time of consent.
- The patient should be warned that further procedures may be required.

Scenario Six

Obese Patients

The major operative difficulties experienced during PCNL in obese patients relate to the length of the body wall track.

The long body wall compromises:

- Needle puncture
- Sheath length
- Intrarenal nephroscope mobility (due to the length of the body wall component of the track)
- Intrarenal access (due to the length of the nephroscope).

Preoperative Planning

CT/IVU

- Measure depth from kidney to skin.
- Entertain alternative treatments (e.g. FURS).

If percutaneous surgery is the only option, the puncture needs to be more vertical.

A vertical puncture reduces the body wall distance.

Nephroscope

Have a "Long" rigid nephroscope and flexible nephroscope (with Holmium laser) available.

Sheath

In an obese patient or a case involving a horseshoe kidney, the conventional Amplatz sheath may only just reach the kidney.

It is very easy, with the increased mobility of the body wall, for the sheath to "disappear" below the skin. It is then extremely difficult (and sometimes almost impossible) to find the sheath.

When a long body wall track is anticipated, obtain a purpose built or prepare a "long sheath" prior to the puncture.

Two other manoeuvres can prevent the proximal end of the Amplatz migrating under the skin.

The first is to fix the sheath to the skin with two large heavy silk sutures.

The second, if using a longer sheath, is to divide either side of the sheath with scissors to skin level, and hold the two flaps created with the tip of artery forceps as for the "peel away" manoeuvre (my preferred manoeuvre) or suture the flaps to the skin.

Should a sheath become displaced under the skin and cannot be retrieved, look in along the guide wire with the nephroscope to the inner lumen of the Amplatz, open the jaws of the alligator forceps distal to the sheath, and gently remove the sheath and nephroscope together.

Alternatively, pass a second guide wire next to the existing wire and thread a Foley catheter over the wire. When the tip is distal to the sheath, inflate the balloon and extract the sheath.

Long sheaths are manufactured but often not routinely available.

The surgeon often needs to create a long sheath. This is easily done as follows:

1. First, place the matching sheath over the dilator. Screw the leading end if a larger Amplatz sheath over the base of the first Amplatz. The outer sheath will now be tightly fixed to the original sheath.
2. Then, measure the distance from the inner aspect of the "crank handle" proximally to the tip of the nephroscope.
3. Cut the sheath to measured length

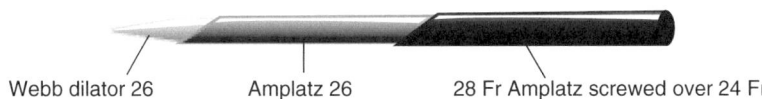

Fig. 6.35 The first step in creating a "long" sheath is to combine two sheaths over a dilator

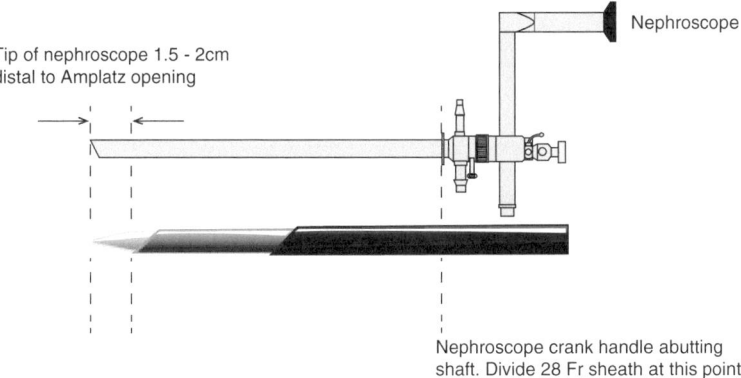

Fig. 6.36 Measure the length of sheath against the nephroscope to allow the distal 1.5–2 cm of endoscope tip to protrude

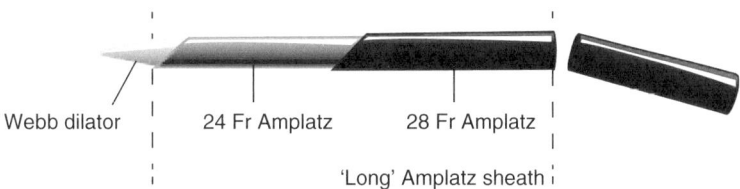

Fig. 6.37 Divide the proximal end of the large sheath proximally at the level of the eyepiece offset with a large scalpel

Scenario Seven

Horseshoe Kidney

Difficulties related to the management of stones in a horseshoe kidney result from the distance of the kidney from the body wall, the complex medial intrarenal anatomy and often poor ureteric drainage. The optimal track entry point is the most upper and lateral calyx as this calyx is "closest" to the skin. However, this calyx is a long distance away and sometimes too far for a rigid endoscope to reach the renal pelvis. Furthermore, even if calculi can be reached, they are commonly inaccessible due to their angulated disposition within the lower medial calyces. Calculi in this situation can usually be visualised and fragmented by a flexible nephroscope and laser fibre. In a horseshoe kidney, the puncture is well away from the supplying vessels and usually bloodless, providing good vision for a flexible instrument. The path from the renal entry to the medial calyces is a gentle curve, which ideally suits the flexible nephroscope and Holmium laser fibre.

It is often stated that the renal blood supply is a potential risk when puncturing a horseshoe kidney. This is not so.

The arterial supply of a horseshoe kidney goes to the medial, inferior and mostly anterior aspect of the kidney. The puncture is lateral and posterior through the most upper and outer calyx, well away from major renal vessels.

The surgeon needs to anticipate the potential difficulties related to a long puncture, compromised medial endoscopic access and potential incomplete stone clearance.

The patient must be warned that stone clearance may be incomplete.

They need to understand that, although the primary aim is to remove all the stones, that is not always possible.

Preoperative Planning

CT–IVU

- Assess the depth of body wall track
- Identify surrounding organs that could be in the path of the needle track (e.g. bowel). Fortunately, this is uncommon.
- Assess the site and nature of calculi. Identify the primary calculi that must be cleared such as stones that are obstructing or mobile in the pelvis and may be causing pain.

Puncture

As this is a long deep track, the puncture needs to be almost vertical into the upper and outer calyx.

Track

A long sheath should be obtained or prepared prior to surgery.

Endoscopy

The surgeon should have long rigid and flexible endoscopes available and a Holmium laser.

Operative Plan

To removal all calculi, but if not possible, to remove those causing obstruction and pain.

Scenario Eight

Large-Impacted Pelviureteric Junction and/or Upper Ureteric Calculus

If these calculi cannot be displaced from below with a guide wire and flushing, and are too large, impacted and hard for ESWL, they can also be extremely difficult to clear by FURS.

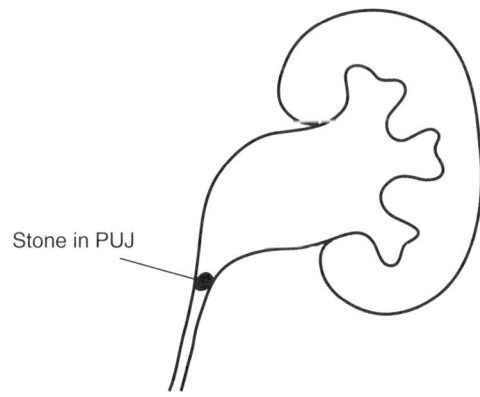

Fig. 6.38 Very large and long-standing calculi are often embedded in the mucosa of the upper ureter

Large Upper Ureteric Calculus

It is always worthwhile attempting to manipulate the calculus back to the kidney – one is often very pleasantly surprised. Once a large stone is replaced into the pelvis, removal is easy by routine PCNL.

If retrograde displacement fails, a percutaneous approach is safe, easy and gives excellent clearance, without damage to the collecting system.

A large, long-standing, impacted (and usually dense) upper ureteric stone can be very tedious or even impossible to remove by FURS.

Plan for Antegrade PCNL to Remove a Large Upper Ureteric Calculus

- The nephroscope needs to enter the upper ureter parallel to its direction, otherwise the ureter tends to angulate medially.
- This angulation compromises access to the stone, and the angled PUJ and upper ureter can catch on stone fragments as they are extracted and traumatise the ureter.
- PUJ trauma can occur unintentionally and undetected during antegrade ureteroscopy from the leading edge of the Amplatz sheath.
- Calculus fragments may migrate down the ureter.
- Consider using the Mini-PCNL instruments which easily enter the ureter from above without damaging the PUJ.

Preoperative Planning

CT–IVP

- Plan the angle for the renal puncture, which will provide the most direct access to the calculus.
- Note the position of the pleura (may need a supracostal puncture to gain the best track angle).
- Confirm the optimal track angle when the patient is in the prone (surgical) position.
- Be prepared to do a "skinny needle" pelvic puncture if the pelvis and calyces above the stone cannot be outlined by contrast.
- Alternatively, be prepared to do a renal puncture using ultrasound guidance and if not familiar with ultrasound imaging, to have a radiological colleague on standby to insert the needle for you.

Fig. 6.39 Renal puncture to access the PUJ should be planned to give direct end-on access to the stone parallel to the direction of the upper ureter

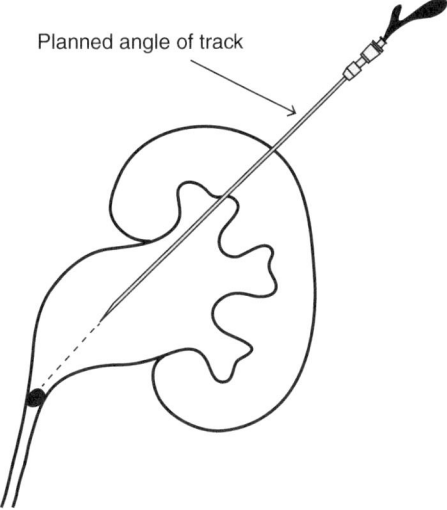

This puncture will usually enter through a mid or upper pole calyx, so the nephroscope and sheath are parallel to the line of the ureter.

- The sonotrode is the preferred lithotrite when a stone is impacted. Broken fragments, which will result from ballistic lithotripsy, can be difficult or unsafe to grasp. The sonotrode will not damage the ureter and aspirates stone particles as it goes.
- Vigorous fragmentation of a calculus tightly impacted in the ureter or pelviureteric junction can result in mucosal or ureteric wall damage – beware.
- Similarly, attempted forced extraction of an impacted stone can traumatise and even dismember the PUJ and ureter.

Procedure

- At the first opportunity, the surgeon should establish a UGW.
- It may be difficult during cystoscopy to manipulate a guide wire and retrograde catheter past the stone. Every effort should be made to place a wire in the renal pelvis, at the time of ureteric catheterisation.
- In my experience, hydrophilic guide wires are the most successful at passing a stone impacted in the upper ureter.
- If the initial ureteric guide wire does not pass the calculus, advance the open-ended ureteric catheter under II until its tip lies just below the calculus.
- Placing the catheter tip next to the stone reduces guide wire buckling and facilitates the greatest amount of forward trajectory for the wire.
- Flushing the catheter with saline may displace the ureteric wall from the stone.
- After flushing, slowly advance the wire towards the kidney.
- If it curls and buckles beneath the stone, withdraw the wire into the catheter.

- Then rapidly advance the wire (like a dart). This is a safe manoeuvre – the wire may pass the stone.
- Straight, floppy-tipped hydrophilic guide wires rarely damage the ureteric wall.
- If the wire moves between the stone and ureteric wall but does not completely pass the stone, advance the catheter tip point to this level using (II screening) and repeat the process of flushing followed by guide wire advancement.
- If no further progress, replace the straight wire with a floppy J tipped wire.
- This may (as described in the management of the complex staghorn – Fig. 6.13) "roll" the wire's leading edge atraumatically between the stone and ureteric wall.
- Provided these manoeuvres are done carefully with hydrophilic wires under II screening, it is very uncommon to cause ureteric damage.
- Should the wire be seen to go outside the ureter on II, further attempts at stone manipulation should cease.
- Should a ureteric catheter pass into the kidney, a renal puncture should be directed through the calyx, which leads most directly and parallel to the upper ureter, usually an upper mid zone or upper pole calyx.
- The aim of the puncture is for the nephrostomy track and nephroscope to enter the kidney parallel to the direction of the ureter.
- Establish a UGW at first opportunity. This straightens the track, reduces the angle made with the ureter at the pelvic ureteric junction and enables the surgeon to employ the "three-wire" antegrade ureteroscopy technique.

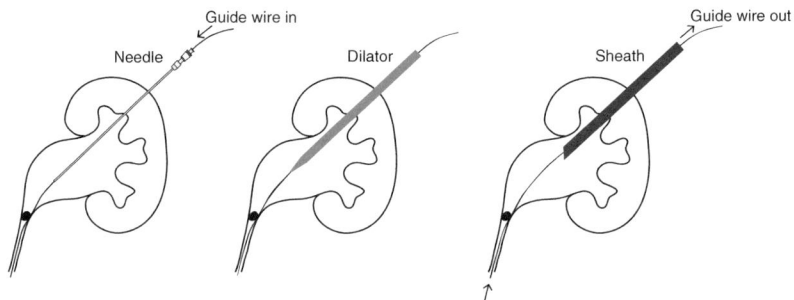

Fig. 6.40 When endoscoping the upper ureter, a UGW is of profound assistance in preventing medial displacement of the ureter and directing the nephroscope to the stone

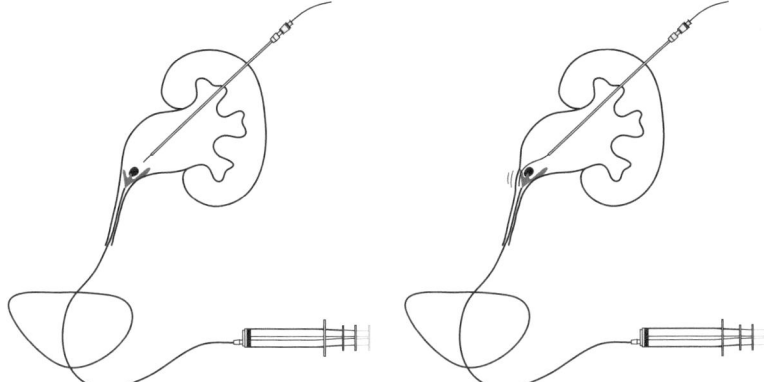

Fig. 6.41 Prior to PCNL, attempt to flush the ureteric calculus into the kidney from below

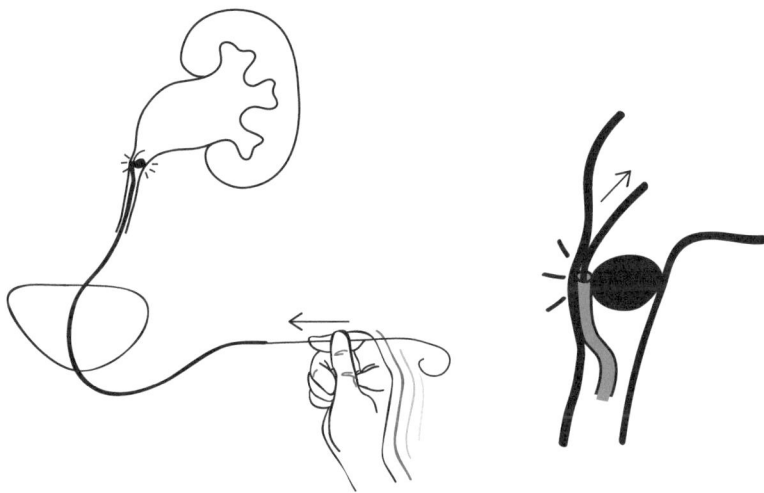

Fig. 6.42 Advancing the straight guide wire from below to bypass the ureteric calculus

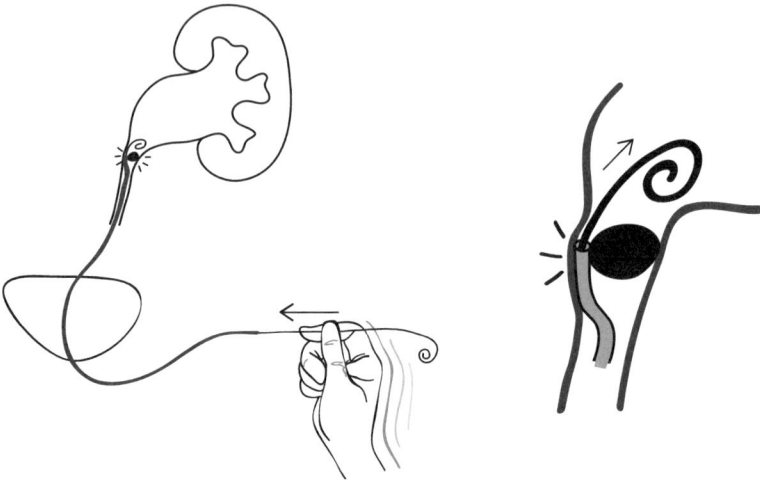

Fig. 6.43 If the straight guide wire fails to pass the stone, replace it with a J-wire, which may "roll" between the stone and the ureteric mucosa

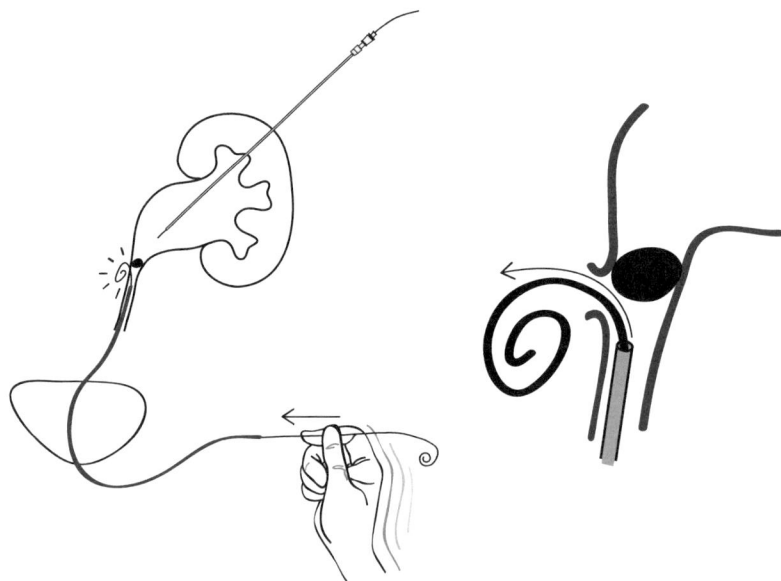

Fig. 6.44 Occasionally, these manoeuvres may perforate the ureter. As the perforation is very small and below the stone, the kidney will not deflate, so the PCNL may still proceed. This will necessitate a "skinny needle" or ultrasound-guided nephrostomy puncture

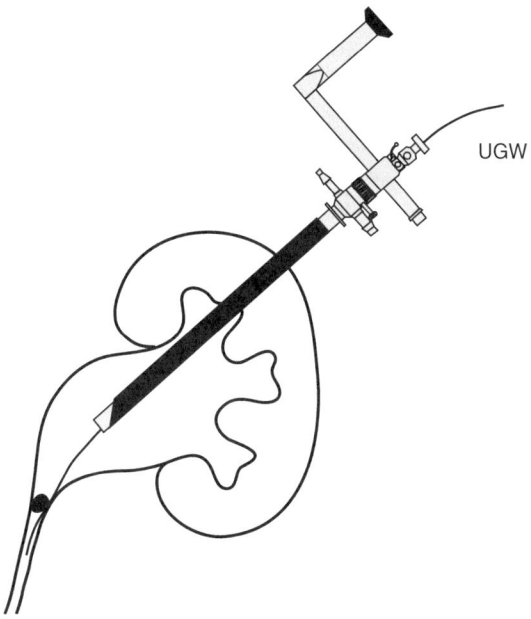

Fig. 6.45 Antegrade ureteroscopy – First establish a UGW

The "Three-Wire" Antegrade Ureteroscopy Technique

The "three-wire" manoeuvre combines a UGW, a separate wire passed down the ureter alongside the UGW and a third GW in the working channel of the nephroscope, which is also passed down the ureter alongside the first two wires. Once the stone is in view, the third guide wire should be removed.

The first two guide wires straighten the track and protect the ureteric mucosa. The third wire leads the nephroscope directly to the stone. When extracting stone fragments from the upper ureter, the sharp edges of the stone fragments often catch on the ureteric mucosa. This can be made worse by the ureter buckling, which can form a flap, as the ureter angles away from the PUJ. The two wires (UGW and second GW) function as a "railway track", straightening this angulation and so allowing the stones to be extracted safely, sliding along and over the two wires, avoiding direct contact with the ureteric mucosa.

Impacted upper ureteric calculi are often large and surrounded by ureteric oedema and ingrowth of mucosa into the surface of the calculus. Many are long-standing and very hard. Removal and fragmentation can be long, difficult and potentially traumatic to the ureter surrounding the stone.

To minimise trauma, wherever possible, fragment and aspirate the calculus fragments using an ultrasonic lithotrite. This reduces trauma and the need to repeatedly extract stone fragments.

I only use the alligator forceps to extract stone fragments from the ureter.

The advancing sharp tines of a triradiate grasper easily perforate and lacerate the ureteric wall and are difficult to disengage from a perforation without tearing the ureteric wall.

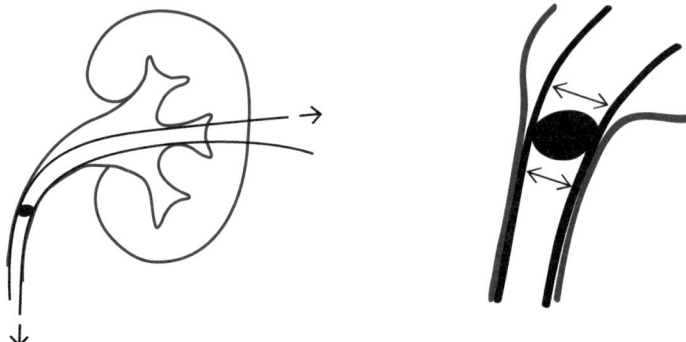

Fig. 6.46 The first 2 of the 3 wires. A UGW is created and a second guide wire is passed through the nephroscope down the ureter

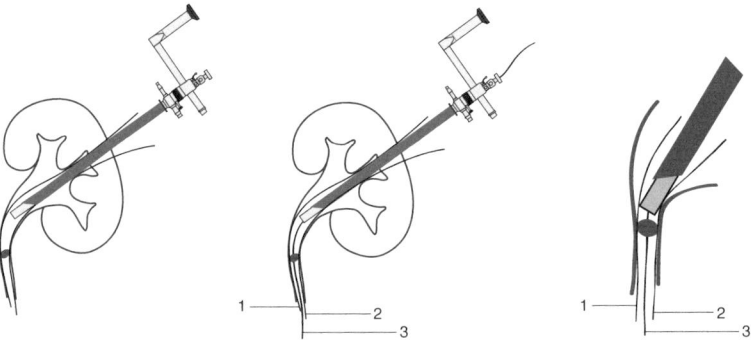

Fig. 6.47 The three guide wires: the UGW, antegrade GW and the third GW in the nephroscope channel

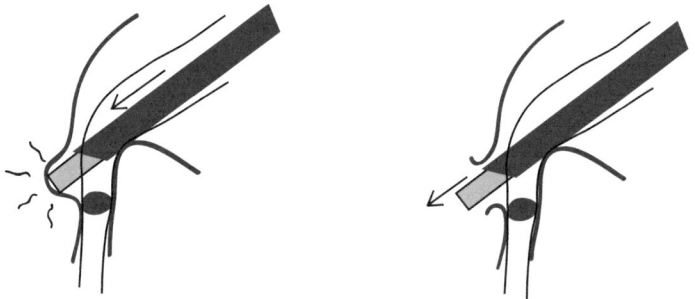

Fig. 6.48 Antegrade ureteroscopy – It is important to pass the endoscope in the line of the lumen of the ureter. Medial movement can damage or perforate the PUJ and upper ureter

Scenario Eight

Amplatz Trauma

When operating in the upper ureter with a rigid endoscope, it is easy for the optical (proximal) end of the nephroscope to "unintentionally" advance the Amplatz sheath.

When looking into the upper ureter, check the proximal end of the Amplatz sheath. If it is in direct contact with the nephroscope, split the sheath.

Displacement of the Amplatz sheath is undetected by the surgeon, because the tip of the nephroscope is 1 ½ – 2 cm in front of the opening of the Amplatz sheath. As a result, the surgeon is "blinded" to inadvertent advancement of the sheath. Being oblique, bevelled and sharp, the leading end of the Amplatz sheath can divide or lacerate the PUJ, behind and outside the surgeon's field of view. This can be avoided by creating a "short sheath", which allows free excursion of the nephroscope into the upper ureter without contact with the proximal end of the Amplatz sheath.

The "short sheath" is fashioned by cutting the Amplatz sheath proximally on opposite sides with scissors and separating the "flaps" by the "peel away" technique (Ref 3.10, 3.11, 3.12).

Following antegrade ureterolithotripsy, a double J stent should be inserted (antegrade or retrograde) and a nephrostomy placed to prevent ureteric stricture formation and facilitate follow-up ureteroscopy if required.

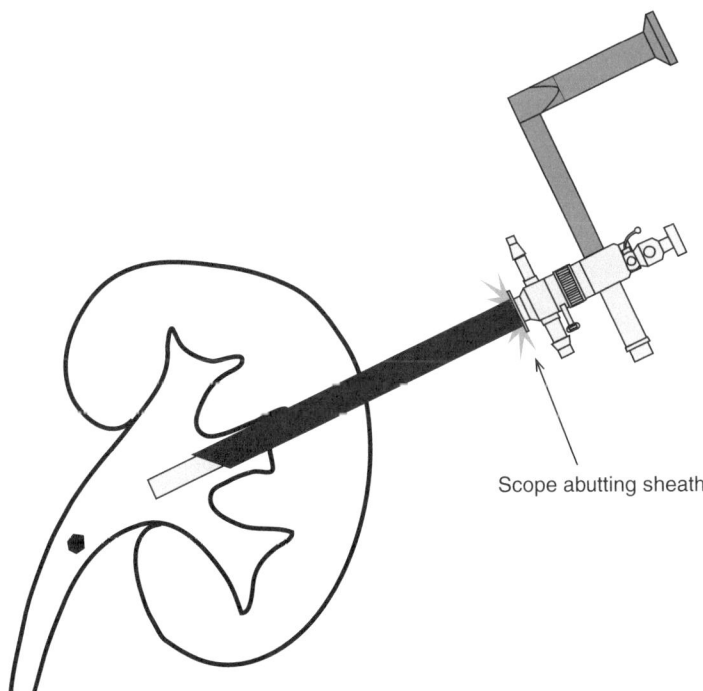

Fig. 6.49 Nephroscope abutting sheath unable to advance

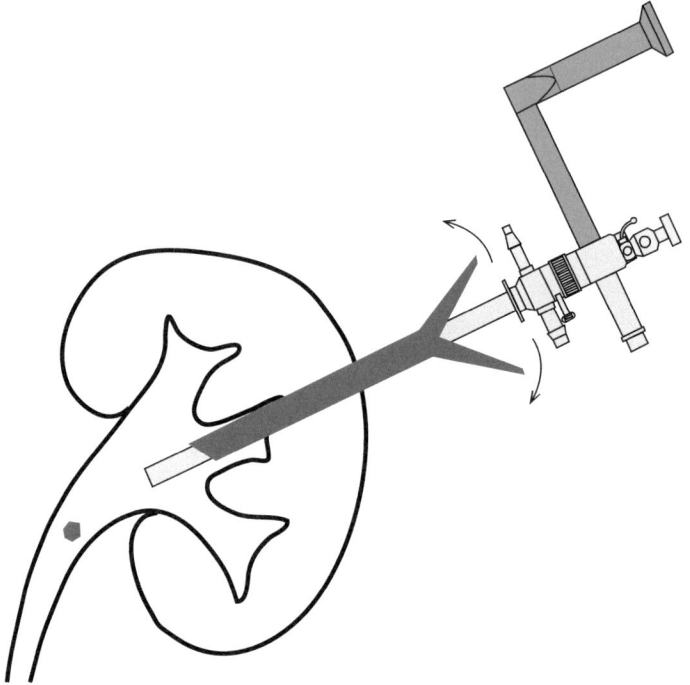

Fig. 6.50 Splitting of sheath to allow nephroscope to advance

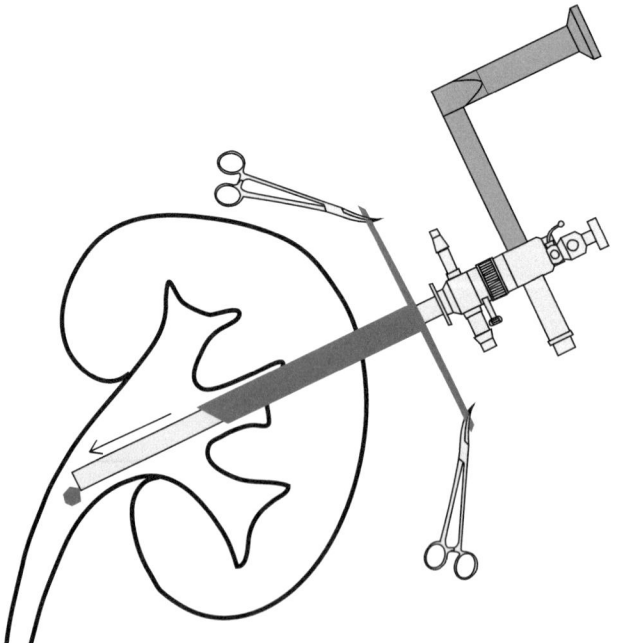

Fig. 6.51 Further excursion of the nephroscope into the upper ureter. (Ref 3.10, 3.11, 3.12)

Scenario Nine

Percutaneous Puncture of a Large Hydronephrosis

There are two potential technical difficulties when puncturing a hydronephrotic kidney. Firstly, deflation of the hydronephrosis. As the kidney is usually thinned, it will collapse before formal dilatation of the track (similar to a suprapubic puncture of the bladder). Secondly, it can be very difficult to radiologically identify a posterior calyx for the needle puncture.

Plan

The aims are to enter the kidney through a calyx and not the pelvis, and to have the dilator and Amplatz sheath well inside the renal pelvis before the hydronephrosis deflates.

Operative Technique

In my experience, the single-stage dilator is optimal for a large hydronephrosis.

Firstly, identify a posterior calyx, if necessary by the air injection technique.

During the insertion of the puncture needle, drain as little urine and contrast as possible to maintain the distension of the kidney.

Do not leave the needle sheath draining freely as this will deflate the hydronephrosis.

Have a guide wire in hand and introduce it as soon as successful entry to the collecting system is confirmed.

The single-stage dilator should be introduced in a single movement. Advance the tip of the dilator to the pelviureteric junction. Insert the Amplatz sheath fully. Only then should the dilator be removed.

Endoscope the kidney immediately and establish a UGW.

By doing this, even if the hydronephrosis collapses, the surgeon can always find the way back into the pelvis, identify the PUJ and place a nephrostomy.

Scenario Ten: Percutaneous Endopyelotomy (Pyeloplasty)

Indications

Endopyelotomy is a "stricture" operation.

The aim of this operation is to divide a stricture that has formed following previous open or laparoscopic pyeloplasty.

In my opinion, endopyelotomy is no longer indicated for the treatment of a primary pelviureteric junction obstructions.

It has been my experience that for an endopyelotomy to be successful, the stricture at the pelviureteric junction must be divided completely to fat, with the division extending ½cm into normal ureter below and renal pelvis above.

If the obstruction appears to "spring open" (in the same manner as division of a bladder neck contracture does following radical prostatectomy), a positive outcome can be anticipated in 70 % of patients.

However, if the stricture does not "spring open", it suggests, there is perirenal and periureteric fibrosis as well as the ureteric stricture, and in my experience these patients do poorly.

In other words, fibrosis external to the ureteric and pelvic serosa cannot be cured by division of the collecting system alone.

As percutaneous endopyelotomy is a "classic stricture" operation, I use a cold knife, and not a diathermy electrode.

If an endoscopic pyeloplasty fails, it is also my experience that to repeat it, is pointless.

Surgical Points of Technique and Difficulties with Percutaneous Endopylotomy

Access

- In a very dilated kidney, the calyces are thinned, so the nephrostomy may enter through an infundibulum or the renal pelvis.
- The trajectory and angle of the puncture and surgery must be calculated so that vision and stricture division are parallel to and in the direction of the ureter.
- Bleeding from segmental or lower pole renal vessels can occur during division of the stricture, so the knife tip must be directed anterolaterally.
- "Bow stringing" of the guide wire through the pelviureteric junction division can displace the PUJ and complicate division.
    - Angulation of the pelviureteric junction away from the division towards the major renal vessels can be exacerbated by pressure from the Amplatz sheath and the nephroscope.

Operative Plan

Previous Surgery

- It is essential to ascertain the technique of the primary pyeloplasty. If it was an Anderson Heinz procedure, the surgeon can be confident that the lower pole vessel will now be behind the obstruction, in other words, between the PUJ and the patient's back.
- Therefore, it will be safe to divide the stricture anteriorly (and so in front of and away from the lower pole artery) and laterally, away from the major renal vessels.

CT–IVP

- Assess parenchymal thickness (assuming a MAG 3 scan has justified the procedure).
- Assess vessel anatomy to exclude large vessels adjacent to the stricture.
- Locate secondary calculi – these must be removed synchronously.

Equipment

- Visual urethrotome (TURP working element and sheath)
- Zero degree cystoscope lens
- Back cutting sickle knife (Storz)
- 6 Fr Double J ureteric stent (to be passed antegrade, does not have to be purpose designed)
- Three straight ahead floppy-tipped hydrophilic guide wires

Percutaneous Puncture

The direction of the track should be planned with the patient in the operative position, so both the track and nephroscopy are parallel to the course of the ureter.

- The puncture should enter a posterior calyx.
- Examine the II-RGP to identify a posterior calyx.
- In a large hydronephrosis, the definition of the calyces may not be clear. The cortex is thin and distended and the contrast is diluted by the large volume of urine in the distended kidney.
- The aim is to enter via a posterior calyx to give:
  - Optimal direction of the percutaneous track
  - Avoid segmental vessels
  - Avoid tearing the renal pelvis
  - Avoid collapse of the kidney with deflation after the puncture and dilation

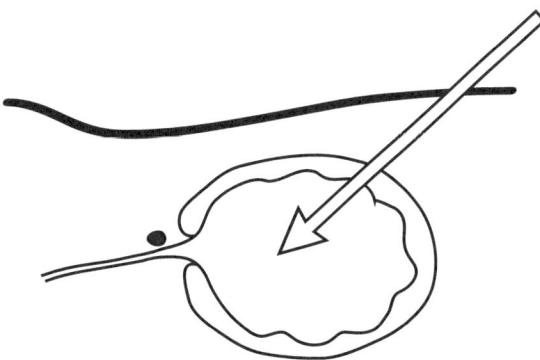

Fig. 6.52 The puncture for endopyelotomy is the same as for access to the upper ureter, as the endopyelotomy incision will be parallel to the direction of the upper ureter

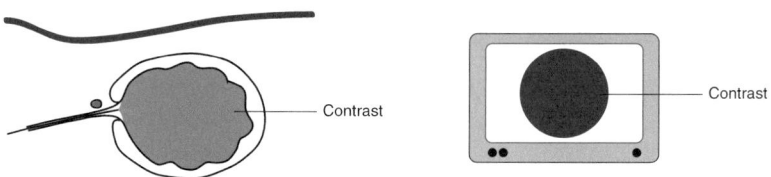

Fig. 6.53 Due to the large volume of contrast in the distended renal pelvis and ballooning of the calyces, it may not be possible to identify a posterior calyx on the monitor

Air Contrast Technique

- Before performing 'air contrast' pyelography, the procedure must be discussed and agreed to by the anaesthetist.
- If it is impossible to define a posterior calyx, the "air contrast" technique can help.
- Air floats. If a small amount of air (2–3 cc) is introduced via the RG catheter during continuous screening, the air will float and accumulate in a posterior calyx.
- The air contrast will outline the calyx to be entered.

The injection of air anywhere in the body is dangerous.

Prior to performing an air contrast study, the procedure should be discussed with the anaesthetist.

Only 2–3 cc of air should be injected through the retrograde catheter. This should be done under II to observe the bubbles as they float and coalesce.

If an attempted air contrast study fails, it should not be repeated.

Once the calyx is identified, the puncture needle should be inserted and the kidney punctured as for a hydronephrosis.

Scenario Ten: Percutaneous Endopyelotomy (Pyeloplasty) 165

Fig. 6.54 The air contrast will often outline a posterior calyx radiologically. Initially, 2–3 ml of air are injected during continuous II monitoring

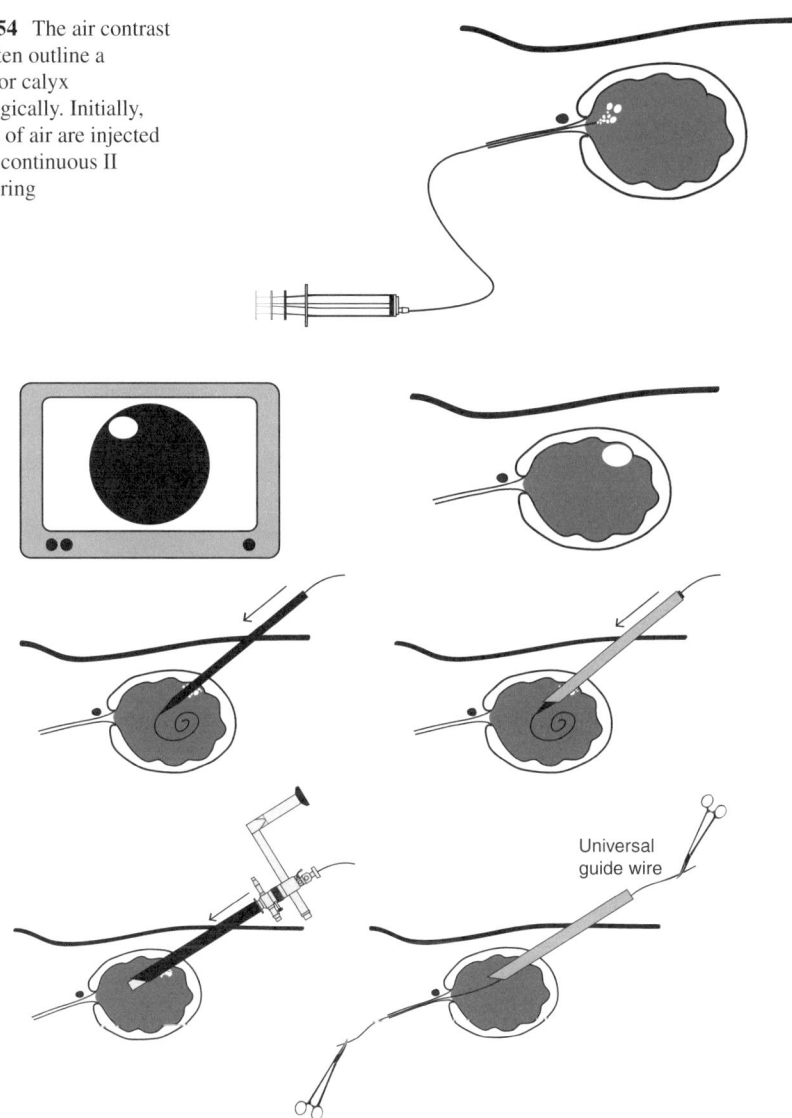

Fig. 6.55 If the bubbles float and coalesce in a posterior calyx, a negative filling defect will appear. This should be punctured and dilated without renal deflation and a UGW established as a first priority

Percutaneous Endopyelotomy: Operative Technique

- The puncture is as described for a hydronephrosis.
- The primary aim is to place an Amplatz sheath into the renal pelvis before it collapses.
- Next establish a UGW. This UGW will identify the lumen of the stricture, straighten the track and prevent medial displacement and angulation of the PUJ and upper ureter.
- Prepare the visual urethrotome using a zero lens and the Storz back cutting sickle knife, before commencing nephroscopy.
- Insert a straight, floppy-tipped hydrophilic guide wire into the visual urethrotome.
- Outside the patient, and before entering the Amplatz sheath, orientate the endoscope so that the sickle knife tip enters the patient in the direction required to cut the stricture, i.e. anteriorly and laterally. I find this very helpful. Once inside the kidney, orientation can become confusing.
- Introduce the visual urethrotome, maintaining the same orientation of the sickle knife blade.
- Pass the second guide wire through the urethrotome and down the ureter to the bladder alongside and parallel to the UGW.
- This will give stability to the PUJ after it is divided and enable the surgeon to control the direction of the ureter, as the wire is coming through the urethrotome alongside the knife.
- Along with the UGW, the second wire straightens the track and prevents angulation of the ureter.
- The second wire along with the UGW also provides a "tram track" for the division of the PUJ, which should be made between the two wires.
- The two wires prevent the PUJ being displaced medially, and spread out, allowing the surgeon to cut between the wires, which support the collecting system on either side, preventing "bow stringing" of the wires through the endopyelotomy.
- The division is performed by gently placing only the very tip of the sickle knife blade between the guide wires.
- The blade is slowly and gently withdrawn towards the surgeon, literally 1–2 mm at a time. This can be done either using the working element operative mechanism, or withdrawing the nephroscope and knife as a single unit.
- It is critical that the surgeon does not take a deep bite.
- The sickle knife is extremely sharp. Being sickle shaped, it behaves like a fish hook and can very easily pick up a large volume of tissue if inserted too deeply, which can be very difficult to disengage.
- The knife should sequentially and slowly divide the stricture until it "springs open". This incision should be continued ½ cm distally into normal ureter, and similarly proximally into the renal pelvis, deep to fat and perirenal tissues.
- It is common to have minor bleeding from the ureteric and pelvic walls during division; this is not of concern and will rapidly settle.
- Following division of the stricture, back load the UGW through the nephroscope using a ureteric catheter.

- Pass a 6 Fr double J stent over the UGW under vision through the urethrotome.
- The stent usually enters the bladder easily through the vesicoureteric junction when it is passed over a UGW.
- Once the stent is confirmed to be in the bladder radiologically, the UGW may be removed under screening.
- I do not routinely leave a nephrostomy.
- However, if the surgeon did wish to leave a nephrostomy because of concerns regarding bleeding or patient stability, it is perfectly reasonable.
- The nephrostomy must subsequently be removed under II screening over a guide wire in the radiology department.
- If not, removal of the nephrostomy may also extract the double J stent, a tedious outcome!

Supracostal Punctures

The only percutaneous route to the kidney is often above a rib.

The most common indications are when treating calculi in an upper pole diverticulum, large staghorn or partial staghorn calculi in the upper pole and mid zone, or in patients with kyphoscoliosis or other musculoskeletal deformities.

Some surgeons access the upper pole electively for the treatment of staghorn calculi.

The relevant anatomy has been discussed previously.

In planning a supra 12 rib puncture, one anticipates potential transgression of the pleura.

However, it is exceedingly rare for the lung to be injured, even in a supra 10th rib puncture.

That said, the surgeon still needs to be aware of the potential for a tension pneumothorax, particularly in patients with severe kyphoscoliosis.

The following potential complications should be anticipated when employing a supra- or intercostal puncture:

- Bleeding from an intercostal vessel
- Pneumothorax complicated by air, blood, irrigant and calculi entering the chest cavity
- Lung injury (exceedingly rare)

Precautions

Bleeding from Intercostal Vessel

Dilate the track immediately above a rib, as the neurovascular bundles run below the rib.

Pneumothorax

- It may be feasible to use a longer track if the puncture is supra 12th rib by starting more laterally, avoiding the pleural reflection.
- Do not use artery forceps to dilate the nephrostomy track for any supracostal puncture, they could tear the pleura.
- Single-stage, balloon or car aerial dilators are ideal if one suspects the track will transgress the pleura as the Amplatz sheath can be inserted without allowing air along the track.
- In contrast, when using serial exchange dilators through the pleura, air can enter the chest between dilations.
- Anticipate a pneumothorax with any supracostal puncture.
- A supracostal approach is an excellent indication for a "tubeless nephrostomy", in which a double J stent is placed at the end of the PCNL, following which the Amplatz sheath is removed quickly during inspiration and the skin puncture immediately closed.
- If there is a large pneumothorax, the surgeon may detect bubbling through the nephrostomy track during the PCNL.
- If one is aware during inspiration that there is a significant or potentially significant transgression of the pleura, before removal of the Amplatz sheath, insert a heavy silk purse string suture into skin around the Amplatz sheath. Remove the sheath quickly, during forced expiration. Immediately cinch and tie the purse string suture. Screen the patient's chest using II in theatre and perform a chest x-ray in recovery. It is very uncommon to need to insert an intercostal catheter. If so, this should be done before the patient leaves the recovery room. A thoracic consult should be obtained.

Chapter 7
Complications of PCNL

Introduction

The kidney is a solid mobile organ with a profuse blood supply and a relatively thin poorly supported collecting system.

Anatomical Factors Related to PCNL Complications

The Kidney

The kidney is a solid fragile organ that easily splits.

The kidney is a pedicled organ, surrounded by fat. As a result, it is very mobile in all directions.

The lower pole of the kidney lies anterior to the upper pole due to its relationship to the psoas muscle behind.

Hence, it is easily displaced forwards by needle puncture, track dilation and endoscopic manipulation.

Following previous surgery or urinary extravasation, the kidney parenchyma, capsule and collecting system can become rigid, fixed and more "brittle".

Hence, previously operated kidneys are harder to dilate and more prone to split and tear during dilation and nephroscopy.

As a result, kidneys that have undergone previous open or percutaneous surgery are more prone to injuries of the collecting system, segmental vessels and parenchyma during PCNL.

Blood Supply

Twenty per cent of the body's circulation flows through the kidneys at the rate of one litre per minute.

The wide bore renal arteries divide anteriorly and posteriorly with the posterior supplying the upper pole. They form segmental arteries before entering the renal substance.

The renal segments or renules are supplied by these segmental end arteries.

Damage to segmental arteries can result in infarction, severe bleeding, pseudoaneurysm or arteriovenous fistulae.

A well-planned radial incision, as used in a nephrotomy, will pass between the segmental supply and is almost bloodless.

Similarly, a properly placed PCNL dilates between segments rather than cutting vessels, so causing minimal renal damage.

The great vessels, e.g. renal vein, IVC, aorta and renal arteries, are in close proximity to the renal hilum and pelvis and so can be damaged during track dilation or nephrolithotomy.

The segmental renal venous drainage, unlike the end arteries, have a cross-circulation. Hence, intrarenal venous injuries are less damaging than arterial injuries.

Collecting System

The collecting system is:

- Only connected to the parenchyma at the fornices.
- Thin and so easily perforated or torn.
- Less supported elsewhere, so the calyces, infundibulae and renal pelvis are all prone to direct damage and tearing.
- Has small volume; the capacity of the average renal pelvis is less than 5 ml.
- Muscular and if irritated, the pelvis and calyces will spasm, making radiological identification of a calyx particularly difficult or impossible in an unobstructed kidney. Hence, many emergency radiological nephrostomies enter through the renal pelvis rather than the tip of the calyx.

Access to the Kidney Is Blind

- The surgeon cannot see the access track, unlike open or laparoscopic surgery.
- This is a "foreign" concept for most urologists.
- The puncture needle, guide wire, dilators and Amplatz sheath are inserted "blindly" using screening alone.
- Radiological imaging is not a familiar skill for most surgeons and requires extensive education, training and practice.

Intrarenal Anatomy

The intrarenal collecting system is small volume and collapses easily, especially when suction is used.

- As a result, it is difficult to aspirate or barbotage blood clot (unlike the capacious bladder).
- The complex angulation of most calyces from the pelvis is greater than the curvature of most flexible nephroscopes.
- As a result of this angulation, irrigation, instrumentation and laser lithotripsy are compromised when using flexible instruments, because the small irrigation and instrument channels are further reduced by angulation of the tip of the flexible nephroscope.
- Consequently, the majority of nephroscopies for PCNL are still performed using rigid endoscopes. These provide optimal irrigation and a straight instrument channel for the deployment of powerful lithotrites and strong stone graspers.
- Although the instruments are rigid, it is my experience that the smaller "mini perc" sheaths have increased intrarenal mobility than larger nephroscopes, particularly when the guide wire is external to the sheath.
- As most calculi treated by PCNL are large and dense, it would seem that rigid nephroscopes are unlikely to be replaced in the near future.
- Because the orientation and direction of the calyces prevent easy access to all areas from a single puncture, complex calculi require multiple access tracks. It is rare to be able to endoscope the entire collecting system from a single track.

Summary

PCNL has many unique potential complications. Most are anatomically based. Serious complications such as bleeding, splitting of the kidney and laceration of the collecting system in particular can occur abruptly.

They can also be anticipated by a history of previous surgery, or anatomical variations seen on the preoperative CT–IVU.

Like TUR prostate, but unlike open and laparoscopic surgery, PCNL is an operation that can be safely terminated and completed at a later date.

Therefore:

- Don't panic or resort to open surgery (unless absolutely indicated, e.g. catastrophic haemorrhage, dismemberment of the ureter).
- Inform the patient during pre-operative consent that the PCNL may be terminated early for medical indications and completed at a later date.
- If PCNL extends for more than 2 h, or surgical complications occur, particularly bleeding not controlled by irrigation, place a nephrostomy and cease the operation.
- Anticipate complications. Have a "battle plan" to avoid and manage complications – each PCNL is unique and should be planned carefully with particular attention to previous history and anatomy of the patient, perirenal structures, the kidney and the stone.
- Always be prepared to return another day.

Complications Related to the Nephrostomy Puncture

Guide Wire Kinking During Dilation

- Avoid!
- I only use hydrophilic guide wires as they do not kink and can be held by artery forceps without damage to the wire.
- However, some surgeons find hydrophilic wire more difficult to control as the wires are slippery to hold and prone to "springing out" if not carefully controlled.
- If using a coiled metal guide wire, it is critical at every stage of the dilation that the dilator and guide wire be parallel with each other to avoid kinking of the guide wire.
- If a metallic guide wire does kink, it is usually very difficult or impossible to continue with the dilation using that wire and so one needs to re-puncture.
- However, it is always worth trying to pass a 6 Fr fascial dilator over the wire. This may enter the kidney and allow the wire to be replaced without re-puncturing.
- Alternatively, sometimes the wire can be advanced under screening so that the kink is inside the kidney or down the ureter – not often successful, but always worth trying before removing the wire.

Damage to Neighbouring Organs

Carefully review the preoperative CT–IVU to plan the puncture, to assess the proximity of neighbouring organs.

Bowel

Generally, the ascending and descending colon lies posterior to the kidney in about one in six patients, most commonly in relation to the left lower pole.

The specific procedures that are most commonly at risk of bowel perforation include the following:–

- Horseshoe kidney (always puncture the lateral upper pole calyx)
- Ectopic kidney
- Kyphosis/scoliosis
- Gastric bypass surgery
- Previous open renal surgery
- Distended colon
- Transplant kidney

Needle Puncture of the Bowel

If one suspects a needle has punctured the bowel, aspirate.

- If gas, it is almost certainly in bowel
- If clear fluid is aspirated, this can be confusing, as it may be small bowel content or urine.
- Infuse contrast and methylene blue through the ureteric catheter in the first instance to determine whether the needle is in the collecting system.
- If no contrast is aspirated after RGS infusion, inject a few millilitres (only) of contrast through the puncture needle under II screening to assess whether it is in bowel.
- If bowel is outlined, insert a guide wire through the needle sheath.
- Leave the guide wire (avoids leaks and helps with the placement of the subsequent calyceal puncture).
- Re-puncture into a calyx.
- Remove the original guide wire.
- A single fine needle puncture of bowel that has not been dilated rarely compromises the PCNL or requires treatment.
- Gas bubbles in the needle or through a nephrostomy track almost always herald a problem, either a bowel or pleural transgression.
- Remember, "bubbles usually mean troubles"!
- Always involve a colorectal colleague if there is suspicion of a bowel injury.

Dilator Trauma to the Bowel

It is possible to complete an uneventful PCNL unaware that the procedure has been performed through a colonic perforation. I find significant bowel injuries are not common, particularly with helical CT, the surgeon should always be prepared for (and can usually avoid) the complication by planning the track or opting for an alternative approach such as FURS. The injury can be diagnosed at various stages:

- During track dilation
- At the end of the PCNL
- Delayed – usually within 24–48 h

During Track Dilation

The colon is mobile and has a tough muscular serosa. As such, the "capsular give" sensation is different when the PCN needle perforates the colon. It seems to require more effort, is prolonged and gives a sensation of "thickness" – difficult to describe but simple to experience. This sensation arouses suspicion.

Usually, the needle has continued through to the targeted calyx, as the puncture is monitored by II. If colon's perforation is unrecognised, then a guide wire is inserted into the kidney and dilators introduced.

If using serial dilators, bubbles may exit from the track between dilators. If so, reinsert the dilator, place an Amplatz sheath, and endoscope the track. I have found that even a small colonic perforation is easily recognisable endoscopically. A cannula can be fed into the colon through the nephroscope and contrast infused to confirm the diagnosis radiologically. My corresponding colorectal surgeons are adamant that firstly, as the perforation is extraperitoneal, it will settle without exploration and secondly, the drain (e.g. Yeates) should be placed alongside the colon, but not through the perforation, to avoid the development of a cutaneous fistula.

At this stage, the PCNL is terminated. If no bubbles appear, one may still be suspicious during dilation, as the dilators often displace rather than perforate the bowel as the bowel musculature is thick. This can be suspected by renal displacement during imaging. The management is the same as for "bubbles", i.e. endoscopy of the track.

Recognition of Perforation at the End of the PCNL

This diagnosis is generally made on the post-PCNL nephrostogram after or when placing the nephrostomy.

The principles of management are to:

- Involve your colorectal colleague.
- Explore the abdomen if there is any suggestion of intraperitoneal leak (e.g. on imaging).
- If the injury appears to be extraperitoneal, separate the bowel and urinary drainage and manage conservatively.

Colonic injuries are rare, variously quoted around at about 1 % of PCNLs.

As a result, experience is limited and so approaches differ. Most agree that a double J stent should be placed into the kidney to create a "tubeless" nephrostomy. The question as to how the bowel diversion is managed I believe should be made by the colorectal surgeon. The team I work with do not favour a tube, such as a Cope nephrostomy, diverting the colon. They prefer a drain alongside the colon. They believe this decreases cutaneous fistulisation from the bowel and assists with closure of the enterotomy. Others recommend a colonic tube. Hence it is essential to have a close working relationship with your corresponding surgeon and manage the patient together.

Should a patient have signs suggestive of peritonitis, intraperitoneal sepsis or prolonged ileus at any time following a PCNL, a significant bowel injury must be suspected and managed in tandem with a colorectal colleague, the usual outcome being laparotomy and proximal diversion of the colon.

Renal Vein or IVC Puncture

- Suspect if you see frank blood from the needle puncture.
- Gently advance the needle sheath and remove the needle.
- Inject contrast and methylene blue via the RGC first.
- If no contrast is aspirated through the needle sheath, gently inject contrast through the needle sheath under II screening, to confirm a venous puncture.
- If only the needle has entered a large vein, the situation is similar to a bowel puncture.
- Leave a guide wire in the vessel; this assists with the direction of the new puncture.
- Puncture into a calyx.
- Remove the original guide wire.
- If a large vein has been dilated or endoscoped, immediately cease the procedure and observe the patient.
- Be aware that if the nephroscope is introduced into the renal vein or IVC, the view of the lumen of large vein scan be remarkably similar to the renal pelvis and calyces.
- As these vascular punctures are usually venous, the patient will usually settle without intervention.
- If a large defect has been caused in a vein wall, such as by a dilator, the procedure should be terminated and the patient observed.

Complications During Track Dilation

- During dilation of the body wall, the dilator may suddenly "jerk" forwards.
- This can split the kidney and perforate the renal pelvis.
- This complication should be avoided firstly by anticipating the potential need for increased force on the dilators (e.g. previous surgery), and secondly, by dilating with the ulnar aspect of dilating hand on the patient's back (Ref: Fig. 5.4), which prevents sudden forward propulsion of a dilator.

Lost Track During Dilation

- Track loss occurs most often when applying force to the dilator to advance through body wall scar following previous surgery.
- Track loss also occurs in a mobile kidney, particularly in the case of a polar puncture (e.g. calyceal diverticulum), as well as in thin patients.
- Should the guide wire be lost from the kidney, remove the needle and wire, realign the direction of the needle parallel to the calyx, and re-puncture.

- Always attempt to manipulate the guide wire down the ureter at the time of puncture – this will give the track stability.
- Commence dilation of the track with fine serial dilators (8, 10 and 12 French – fascial dilators) if the kidney is very mobile.
- This manoeuvre "drills" an initial nephrotomy, allowing the tips of serial or single-stage dilators to enter the parenchyma without pushing the kidney way. This sequence usually prevents renal displacement by larger dilators.
- Insert a "long grey" internal catheter from the Amplatz dilation set.
- This straightens, stiffens and maintains the direction of the track.
- If all of the above procedures fail, insert a 26 Fr dilator over the guide wire and advance the dilator to the outer edge of the kidney.
- Then pass an Amplatz sheath over the dilator to the outer edge of the kidney.
- Once the sheath is in place, remove the dilator but leave the guide wire in the kidney.
- Endoscope the track to the outer border of the kidney (as described in the management of complicated staghorn), and enter the kidney under direct vision using alligator dilators to create an endoscopic nephrotomy (Ref. Figs. 6.16, 6.17, 6.18, and 6.19).
- Then insert a guide wire through the nephroscope under vision into the pelvis and ureter.
- Straighten the kidney on the nephroscope, and if possible, create a UGW.
- It will then be straightforward and safe to dilate the track and clear the stone.

If You Are Unable to Successfully Puncture a Selected Calyx

Use the "Y puncture" technique (Figs. 6.31 and 6.32).

- Puncture a neighbouring calyx.
- Establish a UGW.
- Remove the Amplatz sheath.
- Perform a "Y" puncture into the desired calyx.
- Establish a second UGW and over this track into the targeted calyx.
- Always be familiar with and prepared to use alternative dilator systems, none of the four systems are ideal for all operative scenarios.

Amplatz Trauma

- The Amplatz sheath has a leading edge, which is oblique, bevelled and sharp, and is applied to the Amplatz dilator intimately.
- While advancing the sheath, as long as the leading edge is closely applied to the dilator, it cannot cause trauma.
- However, if the sharp edge extends beyond the shoulder of the dilator, or the dilator is removed and the sheath is advanced without a dilator, the leading edge may lacerate or cut a large core through the kidney or the collecting system.

- It is essential to ensure that the Amplatz sheath and dilator are correctly paired size wise.
- The leading edge of the Amplatz sheath can be unconsciously advanced out of sight by the nephroscope, especially if attempting to enter the upper ureter (Ref: Amplatz trauma and Ref: Figs. 2.10, 2.11, and 2.12).

The Amplatz sheath is not safe if:

- The size of the dilator and sheath are mismatched.
- The leading edge of the sheath advances over the shoulder of the dilator.
- The sheath is advanced in the absence of a dilator.
- The nephroscope is advanced deeply into the upper ureter.

Sites of Amplatz Sheath Trauma

There are three regions at risk of damage:

1. Renal parenchyma
2. Calyceal infundibulum
3. Pelviureteric junction

These complications are all avoidable.

Dilatation

- Only dilate the track and advance the Amplatz sheath under image intensification.
- Watch the leading edge of the Amplatz sheath on II.
- Using a single-stage (Webb) dilator, observe the proximal safety line on the shaft of the dilator.
- Only advance a sheath through the renal parenchyma over a dilator.
- Never advance an Amplatz sheath blind or under II anywhere in the urinary tract if it is not on a dilator.
- The Amplatz sheath may be advanced over a nephroscope in a calyx or the renal pelvis if there is clear 360° view of the tip of the sheath and collecting system.
- Be aware of "unconscious" advancement of the Amplatz sheath by the nephroscope, during antegrade ureteroscopy.
- Advancing the nephroscope into the upper ureter may inadvertently push the sheath forward.
- As a result, the sheath may cut or dismember the pelviureteric junction.

Avoidance of sheath advancement during antegrade ureteroscopy:

- Use a "split sheath" fashioned by the "peel away" technique. This shortens the length of the sheath so that the nephroscope may enter the ureter without impacting on the base of the sheath. (The open phalanges of the split sheath also prevent the sheath being displaced).

Lost Amplatz Sheath

If the Amplatz sheath falls in beneath the skin (particularly in obese patients), it can be very difficult to extract.

This is best avoided in obese patients by making the shortest track possible and securing the sheath to the skin by large silk stay sutures, one on either side of the sheath. Alternatively, the sheath can be cut to form two flaps, which are firmly held externally by an artery forceps on each flap.

To extract the displaced sheath, pass a Foley catheter over the guide wire, inflate the balloon distal to the sheath, which will allow extraction using the balloon.

Alternatively, the guide wire and sheath can be endoscoped, alligator forceps inserted and their jaws opened outside the sheath. Then the sheath can be retracted synchronously with the nephroscope.

One must be careful not to put too much pressure on the jaws of the alligator forceps or the hinge will break.

Forceps Trauma

The most commonly used forceps for PCNL are the alligator and triradiate forceps.

Triradiate Forceps

Features:

- Robust
- Strong grip
- Large fragment extraction
- Fast
- Excellent in the renal pelvis
- Easy to use
- Cheap

The tines of the triradiate grasping forceps:

- Extend away from the scope (reverse action).
- Extend beyond the stone (therefore, out of sight).
- Are sharp.
- Have a "fish hook" tips, sharp and pointing backwards towards the surgeon.
- Should the tines perforate the collecting system, they are extremely difficult to disengage.
- They can tear the collecting system, especially the ureter, during closure or extraction of the forceps.

Prevention of Triradiate Forceps Trauma

- Do not use in the ureter, unless it is very dilated, and the stone edge is well away from the wall.
- Never use blind or under image intensification.
- When grasping a stone, prior to extraction, rotate the forceps.
- This will clarify that neither the stone nor the forceps are attached to or through the wall of the pelvis or ureter.
- If there is any suggestion that the collecting system is perforated by the tines, or the stone is impacted, the surgeon must let go.
- This may be simple.
- However, if there is difficulty releasing the stone, very gently advance and open the tines and extract the forceps open under vision very slowly
- Then, particularly if the stone is impacted, it should be reduced in size by sonotrode lithotripsy.

Renal Pelvis Perforation

This may leak irrigant and stone fragments may extrude.

Management

- If a large defect or rent occurs early in a lengthy stone case, cease and insert a Cope nephrostomy and double J stent.
- If the rent is small, work elsewhere in the kidney.
- At the termination of the procedure, look through the rent and attempt to extract any obvious stone fragments.

Note

- It is very difficult to find calculi once they are outside the kidney. Do not look for them with great vigour, if they cannot be found, they should be left.
- It is exceedingly rare for extravasated stone fragments to require any further treatment.
- It is important to document fragment extravasation, as the opacities can complicate and confuse the interpretation of subsequent imaging.
- Perform a nephrostogram 3–4 days after the procedure. If no leak, remove the nephrostomy over a guide wire in radiology (to avoid inadvertent stent removal).
- Re-endoscopy, usually ureteroscopy, may be performed after 2 weeks.
- Never try to grasp calculi outside the kidney under II with any stone grasper.

Management of a Large Pelvic or Infundibular Tear

- If not already established, create a UGW.
- If the tear is very large, it may not be possible to pass a double J stent, without the upper loop falling outside the rent.
- If possible, a stent and nephrostomy should be inserted.
- If the upper stent loop will not stay in the pelvis, place an antegrade "nephrostent" to the lower ureter and bladder over the UGW.
- If a readymade nephrostent is not available, pass a ureteric catheter from the kidney to the bladder over the UGW.
- Then insert a tube nephrostomy (purpose built, or a whistle tip catheter) over the ureteric catheter so that its tip is seen lying in the renal pelvis on screening.

  Confirm this by nephrostogram.

- Suture the nephrostomy tube to the skin and the RGC to the nephrostomy tube.
- Once the patient's condition has settled, usually after 2–3 days, perform a nephrostogram. If this demonstrates no leakage, insert a double J stent (from above or below), remove the nephrostomy and RGC and leave for at least 6 weeks.
- It is then safe to repeat the percutaneous nephrolithotomy, or if the stone clearance has been sufficient, FURS.

Management of Complete PUJ Avulsion

This is a rare complication but may occur.

Management

- Insert a Cope nephrostomy into the kidney.
- Open the patient, repair and stent the repair.

  Note: I have managed one patient with an avulsed PUJ conservatively with a nephrostomy and stent, only later to have to repair a secondary pelviureteric junction stricture.

Infundibular Tears

These injuries settle without specific treatment.

Sonotrode Trauma

The sonotrode is generally very safe. However, misuse can result in overheating or direct physical trauma.

- It is essential to ensure that irrigation is running through the probe at all times. Otherwise, it will overheat rapidly and the sonotrode generator will "burn out" (expensive and traumatic).
- Beware of "soft" stones, the sonotrode will drill a hole through the stone rather than fragment it.
- As a result, the sonotrode may "bore right through" a large soft calculus very quickly and exit the other side of the stone, out of surgical vision.
- In doing so, the probe can easily perforate the collecting system on either side of the stone without the surgeon's knowledge.

Management

- Be wary.
- Only drill at one site for about half a centimetre, and only while one can see the tip of the sonotrode probe.
- Plan the attack on the stone, "work" the sonotrode, rotating it, and moving sequentially around the periphery of the stone mass.
- Systematically, remove stone fragments as you go.
- If a stone breaks easily, it is usually a layered struvite stone.
- It is very easy to become "over enthusiastic" with the central excavation, and in doing so, leave a mobile outer stone "shell".
- This "shell" of calculus can be frustratingly difficult to fragment, grasp and extract.
- One must have a systemic plan of attack for every variation of stone size, shape and texture when using the sonotrode.

"Lost" Calculi

- After endoscopic clearance of all visible stones, II may demonstrate residual calculi.
- Sometimes, the "calculus" is artefactual and turns out to be contrast contained in a calyceal clot.
- Flush the collecting system through the nephroscope. This may be sufficient to flush away these "opacities".
- If stones are imaged but cannot be seen endoscopically, more than likely they will be in a "parallel lie" situation or a calyx that is too angulated to access from the current track.
- Alternatively, stones may be in the same calyx, but hidden within clot.

Management

- Under screening, withdraw the nephroscope very slowly. When the II suggests the "stone" is at the tip of the nephroscope, slowly withdraw the Amplatz sheath to this level under II screening.
- Then gently grasp or probe the site of the opacity using alligator forceps.
- This will sometimes reveal stone ensconced in clot.

If not, then one has a parallel lie situation.

If that is the situation, management options are to perform either a "Y" or "target" puncture or to leave the stone for treatment at a later date by ESWL, PCNL or FURS.

N.B: Do not attempt to retrieve peripheral or small, difficult stones until all the major central stone mass that is endoscopically visible is cleared. These peripheral fragments usually require considerable angulation and manipulation of the nephroscope, which may start bleeding. They are generally less important to remove than the central stone mass. Prolonged pursuit of these minor stones may precipitate termination of the PCNL, so remove the easy and central stones first and the peripheral stones last.

Similarly, once one embarks on further calyceal punctures, trauma and bleeding may result in rapid termination of the procedure. Hence, it is essential to have cleared all of the endoscopically accessible stones prior to further punctures.

Lost Nephrostomy Track

- If the nephrostomy track is lost, a Cope catheter, Penrose or Yeates drain tube can be placed on the tip of the index finger and pushed down to the perirenal region, to drain the kidney, similar to a standard drain for open surgery.
- Alternatively, or as well, a double J stent is inserted cystoscopically, the "tubeless" nephrostomy.

Urinary Tract Infection and Septicaemia

Management

Pre-operatively

- MSU (remember, a third of patients with sterile urine can have organisms within their calculus)
- We give 48 h of parenteral antibiotic for staghorn calculi prior to PCNL.
- If a diversion or obstruction is associated with infection or a neurogenic bladder, insert a radiological nephrostomy 48 h prior for drainage (this is a great help with access as well) and commence antibiotics after urine cultures are obtained.

Intraoperative Sepsis

- If at the time of the initial puncture, frank pus is aspirated, the procedure should be terminated immediately, a Cope nephrostomy inserted, and an elective PCNL arranged a week or so later following parenteral antibiotics and renal drainage.

Post-operative Fever

- Blood cultures.
- Parenteral broad-spectrum antibiotics.
- Full blood examination and CRP.
- Review – up to a third of patients will have a transient post-operative fever, yet only 1–2 % will turn out to be septic. Until the patient settles and cultures are clear, one has to treat the patient as septic.

If the patient is shocked or hypotensive, transfer immediately to ICU.

Pneumothorax

Suspect a potential pneumothorax in all supracostal punctures, or if "bubbles" occur during surgery or at the time track dilation or the removal of the Amplatz sheath.

- Avoid supra XI punctures.
- A supra 12th rib puncture has a 10 % chance of a pneumothorax.
- If a supracostal puncture is unavoidable:
    - Make the puncture as lateral as possible.
    - Puncture in expiration, to decrease the descent of the pleura.
- A significant pneumothorax is rare.
- The patient's chest should be screened using II on the table at the end of any PCNL involving a puncture above a rib.
- If a significant fluid effusion is seen at the costophrenic angles, it may require drainage.
- A formal chest x-ray must also be performed in recovery for all patients having a supracostal puncture.
- It is unusual to require a chest tube.
- If the pneumothorax is large or there is a suggestion of a tension pneumothorax – arrange an immediate thoracic referral.

Bleeding

- Bleeding can be arterial or venous.
- Venous is rarely a significant problem and settles by tamponade at the end of the PCNL.
- Arterial injuries can result in immediate significant intra- or post-operative bleeding, or delayed bleeding from the development of an arteriovenous fistula or pseudoaneurysm.
- When a fistula develops between an artery and a vein, as the venous pressure rises, it may eventually rupture and bleed.

- Bleeding may be into the collecting system, in which case the patient develops haematuria, or outside, where the urine is clear.
- A pseudoaneurysm damages the arterial wall.
- The vessel will clot and from time to time rupture, from a day to a week or even months after PCNL, resulting in fresh blood in the urine.
- Most operative bleeding is parenchymal, venous and not significant.
- It is controlled by the Amplatz sheath, tamponading the parenchymal segment of the track and irrigation during the PCNL.
- Venous bleeding settles quickly at the termination of the procedure as the kidney returns to its original state, which is a major reason why I use thin Cope nephrostomies that drain urine but not blood through the fine holes, allowing the parenchyma to "collapse" back to normal anatomy, providing tamponade, which stops venous bleeding.
- If a nephrostomy tube is spigotted and this controls venous bleeding, resist any urge to irrigate the nephrostomy if nothing drains after removal of the spigot, as irrigation may dislodge the tamponading clot and reignite the bleeding.
- However, be very wary of heavy bleeding, particularly if vision is lost during irrigation. This is most likely to be arterial.
- If there is a drop in haemoglobin or blood pressure, or the anaesthetist is concerned, insert a nephrostomy, spigot the nephrostomy, terminate the procedure, observe the patient and if necessary, transfer to ICU.
- If there are more than 2 units of blood loss, or continuing blood loss, an urgent angiogram and embolisation is essential.
- Similarly, if a patient presents with a clot retention post PCNL, they must have an angiogram.
- This presentation is usually that of a bleed from an a-v fistula or pseudoaneurysm.
- The general incidence of embolisation following PCNL is about 2 %, but patients with complex calculi requiring many tracks and a long procedure, particularly in the setting of previous surgery, should be warned that their chance is significantly higher. In my own series of large infected Staghorn calculus, most of whom have had previous surgery, the incidence was 6 %.
- If bleeding occurs, 6 weeks to 3 months post-surgery, it is also most likely an arteriovenous fistula or pseudoaneurysm. The patient should be referred for angiography and embolisation.

Residual Calculi

Causes:

- Poor visualisation, e.g. bleeding.
- Parallel lie (inaccessible) calyx.
- Displacement (into the ureter or calyces).

- Early termination of PCNL due to operative complication.
- Elective multistage PCNL.

  Large calculi remaining are best treated by a repeat PCNL.
  Small calculi can be managed by FURS, ESWL or "mini perc".
  If leaving smalls stones, insert a double J stent to facilitate follow-up FURS.
  Planned elective "sandwich therapy" by staged serial PCNL and ESWL does not appear to have stood the test of time as a successful modality for treating larger complex calculi.
  However, the concept of the combination can still be effective in some cases.

DVT

I fit my patients with embolism stockings. DVT post PCNL is rare and the AUA guidelines do not recommend routine DVT prophylaxis in normal patients.

Appendix I: Critical Pathways, Theatre Equipment Lists and Setups

Equipment and Set-Up for PCNL (Nurses Set Up Notes for A/Prof D. Webb Theatre)

Gloves:	8 and 8.5 microthin
Prep:	Betadine

Lithotomy bundle, major bundle, craniotomy drape (in urology room), 3 × gowns, large bowl set

A cystoscopy is done first. A hydrophilic guide wire and 6-Fr ureteric catheter are inserted and taped to an 18-Fr urethral catheter with "sleek" adhesive tape. Patient is then repositioned into the prone position. Surgeon will re-gown.

Note: Have cystoscopy bottom trolley and general top trolley.

Cystoscopy Trolley

- Cystoscopy tray and 30° telescope
- Camera and light lead
- Rubber nipples (grey and white)
- Straight guide wire – Terumo 0.035, hydrophilic, floppy tip
- 6-Fr ureteric catheter (yellow – open ended – Cook)
- 16-Fr two-way Foley catheter and catheter drainage bag
- Raytec gauze × 5
- Single cystoscopy irrigation giving set
- Catheter spigot
- 10 ml- and 20-ml syringe
- Minimum volume extension tubing (140 cm)
- Xylocaine jelly and "sleek" adhesive tape 6″ length doubled at both ends

General Trolley (Top)

- "Bair Hugger" patient warming blanket
- Drape – craniotomy drape (Molnlycke Health Care Ref. 888442)
- General tray
- Camera and light lead
- 25° and 45° nephroscope (both sizes)
- Triradiate grasper (3 prong)
- Alligator grasper
- Scalpel handle and 15 blade
- "Swiss Lithoclast Master" (combined ultrasound and ballistic lithotripsy) – set up and tested
- 23 g injection needle
- Raytec gauze × 5, packs × 5
- 5-, 10- and 20-ml syringes
- Suction tubing (for the sonotrode)
- Double irrigation tubing (for saline irrigation)
- 3 straight floppy tipped "hydrophilic guide wires" – (as for cystoscopy)
- One "J"-wire
- Cook nephrostomy sheathed needle (urology room –19 g 19 cm)
- Webb single-stage dilators, size 26 and 28 Fr with appropriate Amplatz sheaths
- Cook Amplatz sheath dilator set (do not open; only used if there is difficulty with Webb dilator insertion)
- "Long grey" Cook internal catheter for use with Amplatz renal dilator set – Cook 8.0 Fr (urology room)
- Grey fascial dilators (8, 10, 12 Fr in urology room – Cook), Omnipaque 350/50 ml mixed
- 50/50 water (n/saline 0.9 %)
- Methylene blue – 1 ml

Drains and Dressings

(NB: Have the PCN needle, 15 scalpel blade, one artery forceps and a 5-ml syringe available in a separate kidney dish for Prof Webb to access.)

- Cook-Cope loop nephrostomy catheters (10 and 12 Fr) (Cook – Multipurpose Drainage Catheter – Ref: 907273)
- Coloplast drainage bag (300 ml)
- 0.9 % saline for irrigation (warm) 10 and 2 l bags
- Needle holder
- Dissector – Gillies
- Silk on cutting edge needle (C17 – 75 cm)

For Endoscopic Pyeloplasty/Endopyelotomy

Add:

- Optical urethrotome tray
- Urology 0° 5-mm telescope
- Optical urethrotome sheath and working element
- Stortz cold "back cutting sickle knife"

Subtract:

- Sonotrode and lithoclast (unless calculi also present – check with surgeon)

Positioning for Patients with Skeletal Deformities and Spinal Cord Injury

- Olympic Vac-Pac (vinyl bags with plastic beads which mould to the patient shape after vacuum suction) – size 31

Nurse Information for PCNL

This information is provided to nurses starting in the PCNL theatre.

Information Sheet

There are two stages to the operation.

Stage 1: Cystoscopy

Is for the placement of a ureteric catheter (yellow ureteric catheter) via the urethra into the pelvis of the kidney. This catheter is used to inject contrast, coloured with blue dye into the kidney during the PCNL procedure (stage 2). This catheter is introduced via rigid cystoscopy, a guide wire is passed through a double bridge, and the yellow catheter is threaded over the wire under image intensification. When the catheter is in place, it is secured to a urethral Foley catheter with 1-in. sleek waterproof tape. A sterile cap is placed on the yellow catheter connector to retain sterility while positioning the patient for stage II.

A/Prof Webb will always use a 6-Fr ureteric catheter and the Albarran deflecting mechanism.

The ureteric catheter is placed through the Albarran into the ureteric orifice, and then the guide wire is threaded through the inside of the ureteric catheter. The ureteric catheter and cystoscope are then removed and yellow catheter positioned over the guide wire to the renal pelvis.

Stage 2: Kidney Puncture and Removal of Stone

(Patient lying prone) The patient is positioned prone on pillows.

The patient is taken from lithotomy (in Stage 1) and placed back on the trolley. Many hands are required to transfer the patient from the trolley to the operating table (prone)

The PCNL equipment is placed opposite the surgeon at the foot of the bed on the surgeon's side.

The theatre technician will oversee the connection of tubing from the ultrasound (sonotrode) from drape to the sucker bottle and the tubing handpiece (sterile) to the lithoclast generator.

Normal saline (warm) is used for irrigation. Ten bags should be available in the warming cabinet.

The II (X-ray) machine is constantly used during this stage. The "C-arm" comes under and over the operating table from the side opposite the surgeon.

At the start of the case, it will be quite hectic as all equipment, nephroscope, light leads, irrigation tubing, camera, sonotrode and lithoclast are passed off to be connected.

The ultrasound lithotripter handpiece needs to be primed by placing the tip in a bowl of water and pressing down on foot pedal until fluid can be seen to be sucked up by the sucker tubing.

Contrast: 50:50 n/saline and Omnipaque 350 mixture with a few drops of methylene blue used throughout

A puncture is made into the kidney using the nephrostomy (Cook) needle. An artery forceps is used under II to gain direction and assist the surgeon with placement of the needle.

Drawing back fluid through a 3-ml syringe will hopefully produce blue-coloured urine from the kidney.

A guide wire is then placed though the needle sheath and dilatation will commence. This is necessary for the nephroscope to be placed: a hole enabling the 24-Fr scope to be placed needs to be made.

Dilatation can be varied; however, normally one of two procedures takes place.

1. Puncture needle, guide wire, Webb SSD (ask which size needed) – (one stage dilatation)
2. Puncture needle, guide wire, fascial dilator, long grey dilator, blue Amplatz dilator (ask which size) – (multistage dilatation)

The ultrasound (lithotripter) is used for softer stones and the lithoclast (jack hammer) for harder stones.

Once the stone has been broken into smaller fragments, it will be removed with either the triradiate or alligator forceps. These stones may or may not be sent to biochemistry or pathology for stone analysis or culture.

At the end of the case, a Cope nephrostomy tube will be left in situ, sizes range from 10 Fr to 14 Fr which are sutured in with silk through the skin edge.

A sterile wafer and non-sterile bag are placed over the nephrostomy tube.

Post-operative Patient Instructions

Going Home After Your PCNL

Discharge information:

This handout includes important information for you to follow when you leave the hospital after your PCNL (percutaneous nephrolithotomy). It is not intended to replace discussion with your doctor, nurse or other members of your health-care team.

Before you leave the hospital, a nurse will talk to you about what you need to do when you go home. If there is anything that you don't understand, *don't be afraid to ask*.

Your *local doctor* will be told when you leave the hospital and they can also answer your questions and provide care and support.

Comfort and Pain

You may notice a burning sensation when passing urine, this is normal and may persist for a few days. This can be relieved by taking Ural sachets four times a day or as directed by the doctor. Ural decreases the acidity level in your urine, therefore reducing the burning sensation you may feel when urinating. Paracetamol (analgesia) may also help. You may also notice your urine colour is blood stained or has some clots in it. This is normal after your procedure and should be clear after a few days.

Dressing

You may have a small gauze dressing to catch any discharge from the wound on your back. The dressing will be changed before you go home if needed. Remove the dressing in 2–3 days' time and leave exposed. See your local doctor if you have any concerns about your dressing or wound.

Medications

Take your medications as instructed by the pharmacist or your doctor. If you were taking blood thinning medications, recommence it 7 days after your operation, unless otherwise instructed by your doctor.

If you are not clear on how and when to take your medications, make sure you ask the pharmacist or doctor before you leave hospital.

Activity

Avoid doing any heavy lifting, straining or strenuous exercise (e.g. lawn mowing, bowling or jogging) for at least 4 weeks after your operation or until you have had your review appointment.

Hygiene

Drink at least 1 ½–2 l of fluid each day (that's about 6–8 of 250-ml glasses), unless you are on fluid restriction. This is important to help cleanse (flush out) your urinary system.

Nutrition

Eat a high-fibre diet to avoid constipation.

Returning to Work and Driving

Avoid operating heavy machinery for at least 4 weeks after your operation. Discuss your individual situation with your doctor as to when to return to work. If you require a medical certificate, please ask your doctor before going home.

If problems arise:
If you experience any of the following after you return home:

- Fever or chills
- Wound swelling, weeping or redness
- Difficulty passing urine
- Inability passing urine
- Fresh blood or excessive old blood or clots in your urine
- Excessive or constant pain that is not relieved with regular pain medications

Or, if you have any other concerns, contact the urology registrar at the Austin Hospital or your local doctor. If you are unable to contact your local doctor, come back to the Austin Health Emergency Department or go to your nearest available emergency department.

Your review appointment:

A follow-up appointment with the urology department will be made and given to you by the ward clerk before going home. If you are unable to receive your appointment on the day of discharge, it will be sent to you by post.

If you are a private patient, you need to contact your private doctor's rooms for a follow-up appointment after discharge.

Consent Form

A standard PCNL usually requires hospitalisation for 2–5 days after the procedure. The urologist may order additional imaging studies to determine whether any fragments of stones are still present. These can be removed with a nephroscope if necessary. The nephrostomy tube is then removed and the incision covered with a bandage. The patient will be given instructions for changing the bandage at home.

The patient is given fluids intravenously for 1–2 days after surgery. Later, he or she is encouraged to drink large quantities of fluid in order to produce about 2 l of urine per day. Some blood in the urine is normal for several days after PCNL. Blood and urine samples may be taken for laboratory analysis of specific risk factors for calculus formation.

Risks

There are a number or risks associated PCNL:

- Inability to make a track to insert the nephroscope. In this case, the procedure may be converted to open kidney surgery or ceased to try an alternative at a later date.
- Bleeding: bleeding may result from injury to blood vessels within the kidney as well as from blood vessels in the area of the incision. 1–2 % of patients may require a blood transfusion or X-ray procedure to stop ongoing bleeding.
- Infection in the urine or blood.
- Fever: running a slight temperature (101.5° F: 38.5° C) is common for 1 or 2 days after the procedure. A high fever or a fever lasting longer than 2 days may indicate infection, however, and should be reported to the doctor at once.
- Formation of an *arteriovenous fistula*: An arteriovenous fistula is a connection between an artery and a vein in which blood flows directly from the artery into the vein. These can take weeks or months to form and can cause bleeding into the urine.

- Need for retreatment: In general, PCNL has a higher success rate of stone removal than extracorporeal shock wave *lithotripsy* (ESWL). PCNL is considered particularly effective for removing stones larger than 3 cm. and staghorn calculi. Retreatment is occasionally necessary, however, in cases involving very large stones.
- This can be by ESWL, redo PCNL or ureteroscopy.
- Injury to surrounding organs: in rare cases, PCNL has resulted in damage to the spleen, liver, lung, pancreas or gallbladder.

Normal Results

PCNL has a high rate of success for stone removal (over 96 %).

Appendix II: PCNL Workshop

This PCNL workshop has been presented and modified over 30 years in Europe, Asia and Australia. It is simple to set up in any urology department, does not require any equipment that would not already be readily available in a hospital performing endourology. As there is no need for any reusable equipment such as nephroscopes or lithotrites to have contact with cadaver or animal tissues, standard theatre instruments can be used for this workshop.

I recommend that the workshop manual be forwarded to participants in advance for preliminary familiarisation.

East workstation requires an experienced demonstrator.

I find that four to six participants can comfortably attend each workstation simultaneously and that each workstation can be completed easily in 15 min.

I recommend a short introductory presentation on PCNL in general and an outline of aims of the workshop.

Participants should spend 15 min at each workstation.

A 15-min tea break mid-workshop provides a timely break for discussion. We always incorporate the "trade" (i.e. endoscope, lithotrite, stent, dilator, needle and guide wire manufactures and imaging companies) to attend as participants and demonstrators. They enjoy the surgical instruction, provide excellent information to our urologists regarding the features and application of their products and have the opportunity to display their wares.

Workstations

Workstation 1:
The surgical anatomy of the kidney and collecting system for PCNL.

Workstation 2:
Techniques and equipment required to create a routine PCNL track.
Workstation 3:
Difficult renal punctures and access.
Workstation 4:
Renal trauma from PCNL access and how to avoid it.
Workstation 5:
Equipment for percutaneous endoscopy, stone fragmentation and stone extraction.

Participants

Divide into groups of 2–3 depending on numbers. Two groups for each workstation per 15 min rotation

Materials Required for This Workshop

1. Porcine kidneys
    Complete with their renal pelvis (and if possible with the upper ureter attached). It does not matter if the renal pelvis of the kidneys have been "slashed" when slaughtered (two kidneys for workstations 1, 2, 3 and 4 per rotation of participants, e.g. 36 participants = total of 48 kidneys).
2. Guide wires:
    (a) Hydrophilic or "slippery" guide wires (straight and floppy tipped)
       ($\times$ 20 – workstations 1, 2, 3, 4 and 5)
    (b) Coiled metallic guide wires
       ($\times$ 6 – workstation 2)
    (c) "J-wire" (all with "Golf Tee" introducers)
       ($\times$ 6 – workstation 2)
3. Large scalpel ($\times$ 4 – workstations 1, 2, 3 and 4)
4. Heavy "nurses'" scissors ($\times$ 2 workstations 2 and 5)
5. Gillies dissectors (or equivalent) ($\times$ 2 – workstation 1)
6. Straight artery forceps ($\times$ 8 – workstations 2, 3 and 5)
7. Percutaneous puncture needles complete with outer sheath ($\times$ 10 – workstations 2 and 3)
8. Renal dilator with Amplatz sheath ($\times$ 3 sets – workstations 2, 3 and 4)

    (a) Serial Amplatz dilators
    (b) Balloon system dilators
    (c) Metal telescoping dilators
    (d) Single-stage dilators (Webb)

9. Amplatz sheaths ($\times$ 2 extra – workstation 5)

Equipment for Workshop 5

1. Stone graspers: (× 1 set)

   (a) "Alligator" forceps
   (b) "Triradiate" forceps

2. Ureteric baskets (assortment)
3. Cope loop nephrostomy (12 French)
4. Stone "dummies" (chalk) (× 1 packet)
5. 2 glass beakers and water (for endoscopic stone fragmentation and ex situ nephroscopy)
6. Nephroscopes:

   (a) Rigid nephroscopes

      (i) "Crank handle" 90° offset lens or
      (ii) 30° offset rigid nephroscope or both

   (b) Flexible nephroscope

7. Endourology equipment stack and shelves:

   (a) Light source
   (b) Camera
   (c) Video system and screen

8. Saline irrigation
9. Lithotrites:

   (a) Ultrasonic probe (sonotrode) including:

      1. Pedal
      2. Power box
      3. Suction
      4. Saline irrigation

   (b) Pneumatic lithotrite lithoclast including:

      1. Power box
      2. Gas cylinder
      3. Foot pedal

Stations

Station 1: The Surgical Anatomy of the Kidney and Collecting System Related to Percutaneous Renal Surgery (PCRS)

Equipment Required

Large porcine kidneys, two per group

Gillies dissectors, large knife or scalpel
Hydrophilic guide wire with stiff proximal end

Aims

To understand the surgical anatomy of the kidney, vessels and collecting system related to PCRS.

Observations

Kidney

1. Renal capsule:
    Note that this is tough, adherent to the outer parenchyma and more resistant and tougher than the parenchyma.
2. Renal parenchyma:
    Note that the parenchyma is narrowest at the tips of the calyces and thickest at the tip of the pyramids.
3. Renal sinus:
    Note that the renal sinus is the space between the collecting system and parenchyma. This extends medially from the outer aspect of the calyx (fornices), along the infundibulum, and becomes progressively larger between the renal pelvis and kidney.
    Note that this space contains fat and the segmental vessels. There are no vessels within the lumen of the collecting system.
4. Collecting system:
    Note that the renal collecting system is only attached to the kidney at the tip of the papilla and fornices. Otherwise, the infundibulum, pelvis, ureter and pelviureteric junction are unsupported and mobile.
5. Pelviureteric junction:
    Note the sudden narrowing and funnelling of the pelvis at the pelviureteric junction to become the upper ureter.

Tasks

Using dissecting forceps indent the capsule noting its resistance as the kidney "dimples" (Fig. 1).

Then grasp and tear the capsule noting its adherence and strength (Fig. 2).

Pass a guide wire, "stiff end" first (i.e. proximal end) up to the ureter and push the stiff end out through the outer border of the kidney (Fig. 3).

Along this guide wire, make longitudinal section (bivalve) of the kidney over the guide wire. This will display the collecting system (Fig. 4).

Fig. 1 Indent and grasp capsule

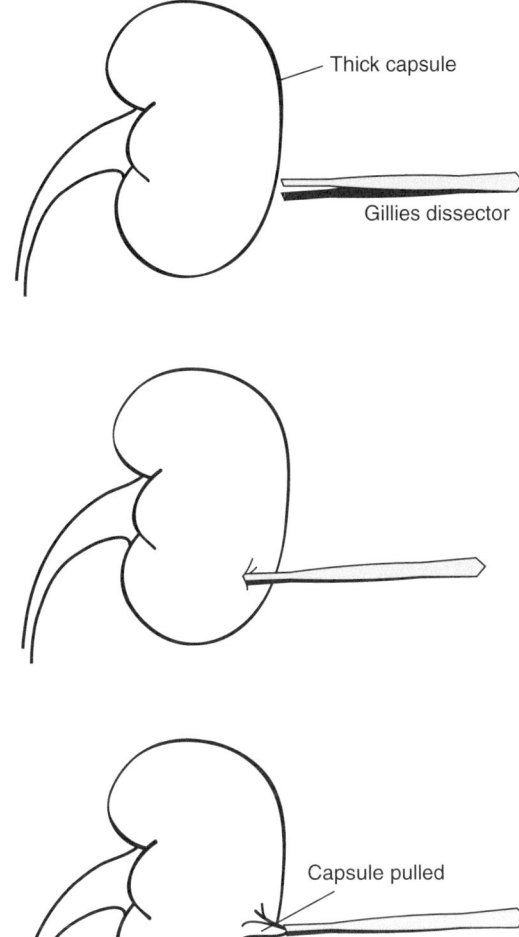

Fig. 2 Retract and tear capsule

Using the Gillies dissectors, pull on the calyceal infundibulum. Demonstrate that the infundibulum is free and mobile and that the attachment of the collecting system is only at the tip of the calyx and the fornices (Fig. 5).

Note that the infundibulum of the calyx may narrow before it joins the pelvis.

Note that the pelvis, pelviureteric junction and ureter are freely mobile and unsupported. The fat and major renal vessels run in the renal sinus.

Cut through the pelviureteric junction over a guide wire, note that it is thick and narrow.

Cut the second kidney horizontally in a guillotine fashion where the wire exits (Fig. 6).

Observe that the calyces have an anterior and posterior disposition. Usually one calyx is more lateral than the other (but this is inconsistent) (Fig. 7).

Fig. 3 Pass the ureteric guide wire out through the capsule

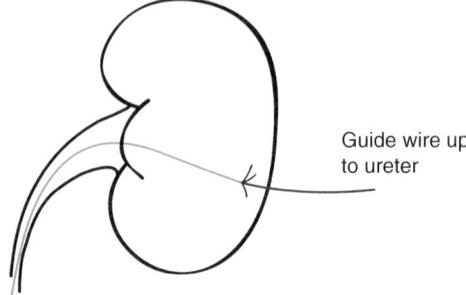

Fig. 4 Bi-valved kidney (vertical)

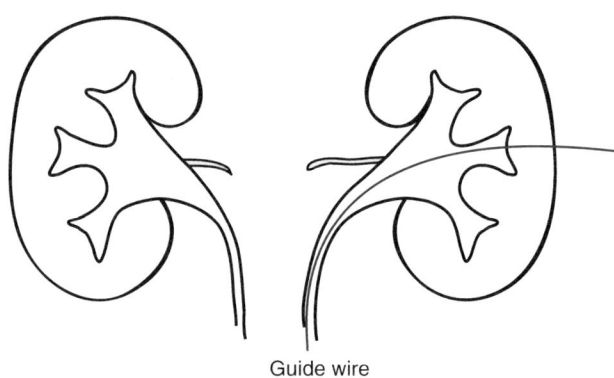

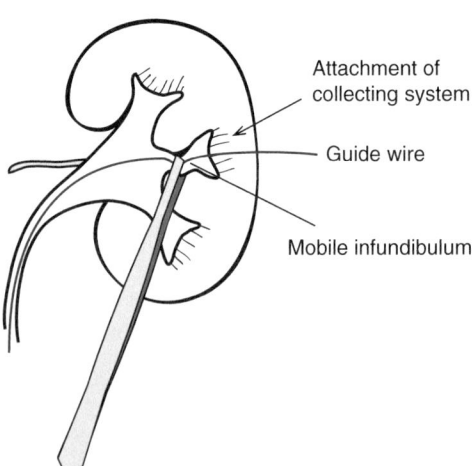

Fig. 5 Grasp and pull the infundibulum to appreciates its mobility

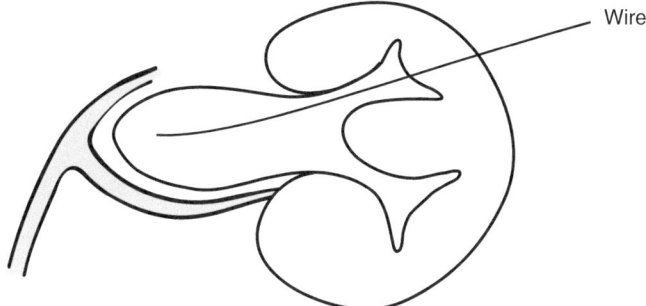

Fig. 6 Transverse section of the kidney

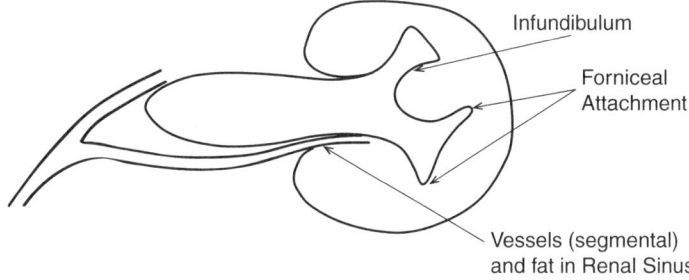

Fig. 7 Anatomy of the transverse section

Repeat the examination of the forniceal attachments and the mobility of infundibulum and collecting system as for the vertical renal section.

Station 2: The Surgical Anatomy of the Kidney and Collecting System Relating to the Establishment of a PCRS Track

Equipment Required

Guide wires, metallic and hydrophilic
    Percutaneous puncture needles and sheaths
    Renal dilators (Amplatz serial, car aerial, balloon, single stage)
    Amplatz sheaths
    Straight – artery forceps (three)
    Porcine kidneys (two per participant)
    Scissors

Aims

1. To familiarise the surgeon with the functions and characteristics of the wide variety of access needles, guide wires, and renal dilatation system and Amplatz sheathes.
2. Illustrate the techniques of making a routine PCNL track with each of the above systems.

Observations

Guide Wires

Observe the different types of guide wires:

(a) Solid core guide wires (slippery and hydrophilic).
(b) Metallic coil guide wires.
(c) Note the variety of wire tips, straight ahead, slightly angled or "J" shaped.

Note the stiff proximal end of most guide wires. If this end is introduced instead of the floppy end, it may perforate the kidney, ureter, or renal pelvis.

Observe the "frictionless" or "slippery" characteristic of the hydrophilic guide wires when wet.

Note their innate springiness. This feature, in combination with their lack of friction or "slipperiness", may result in the wire falling or springing out of the PCNL needle sheath or the collecting system if the wire is not carefully held by artery forceps during PCNL.

Note that even with extreme bending and manipulation, solid core hydrophilic guide wires do not kink.

Compare this to the coiled metallic guide wires, which kink easily, preventing the subsequent advancement of dilators or needle sheaths over the wires.

Note the tolerance of a hydrophilic wire to clamping with artery forceps, which may be used to hold hydrophilic guide wires.

Artery forceps will not damage hydrophilic guide wires but will crush and kink coiled metallic guide wires, rendering them unworkable.

"J"-Wires

Note how the "J" shape forms when the tip of the "J" line is advanced through the tip of the "Golf Tee" introducer. Advancement of the wire occurs at the leading curved edge rather than the tip. This atraumatic curve can be manipulated to advance the wire between a stone and the collecting system (Fig. 8).

Appendix II: PCNL Workshop

Fig. 8 The technique of introducing a "J" wire into a straight needle or sheath

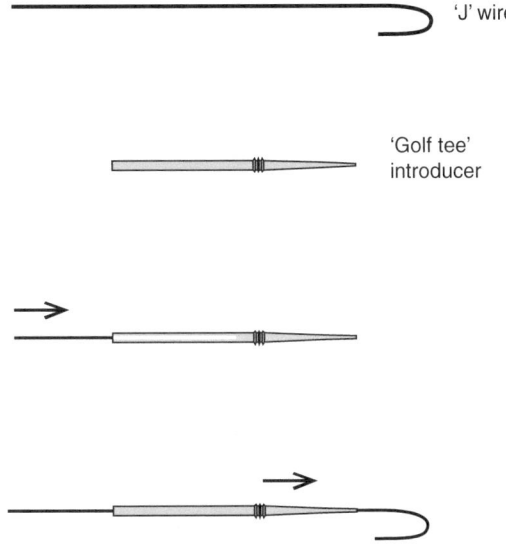

Needles

Observe the needle tips. They can be "diamond" or bevelled in taper (Fig. 9).

The tapered tip moves directly ahead. A bevelled tip may deviate towards the leading edge of the bevel (Fig. 10).

The bevel can be used to advantage, to curve the needle track when puncturing the kidney.

The direction of the bevel is marked on the hub of the stylet of the needle externally, to guide the surgeon or radiologist.

Inspect the transparent outer sheath. Note that the tip of the sheath is slightly bevelled. It is thin and less robust at this point.

This tapering may result in the tip of the sheath becoming scuffed and damaged, particularly when penetrating the skin.

The skin must always be punctured through to fat using a small fine scalpel before introducing the needle, to avoid damage to the sheath.

The sheath is transparent, so that aspirated blood, urine and methylene blue dye can be seen.

Only a very small volume (<1 ml) of fluid needs to be aspirated to be visually apparent.

Note the proximal Luer lock on the outer sheath. It serves as a funnel to insert guide wires and to attach syringes and tubing.

Note that it can be difficult to insert a guide wire directly into the sheath via the Luer lock. The "Golf T" introducer facilitates insertion of the guide wire into the needle sheath (Fig. 11).

Needles are strong. They are made of springy steel, which can be flexed to alter the direction of the needle tip by the surgeon.

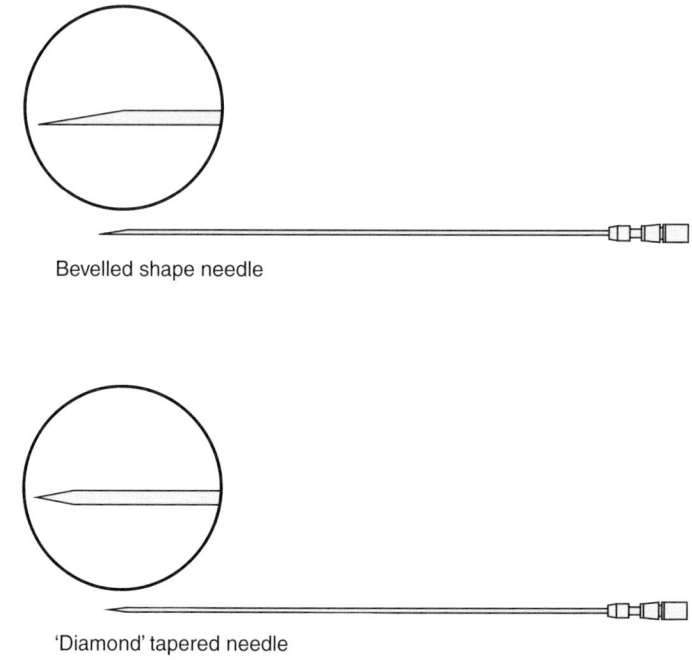

Fig. 9 Puncture needle tip options

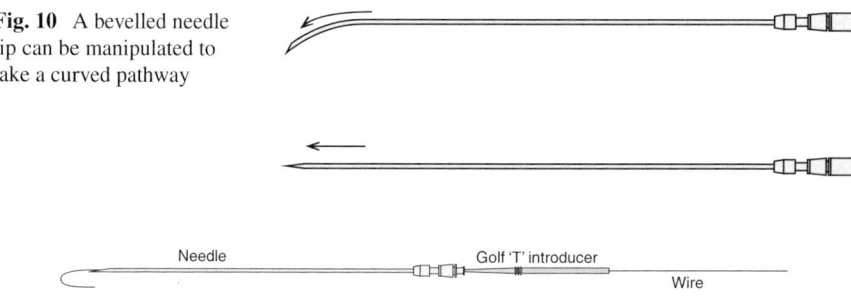

Fig. 10 A bevelled needle tip can be manipulated to take a curved pathway

Fig. 11 Method for introducing a curved 'J' wire into a straight needle

Dilators

Amplatz Dilators

These are serial fascial dilators.
   The first step in dilatation is a needle puncture of the kidney and insertion of a guide wire (Fig. 12).

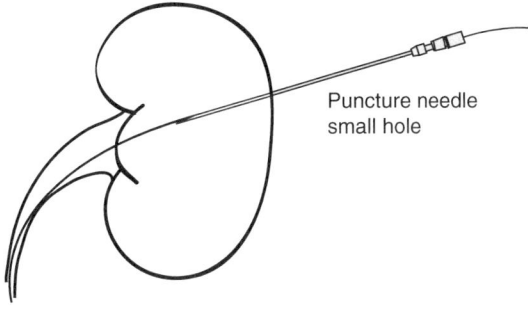

Fig. 12 Renal needle puncture and introduction of a guide wire

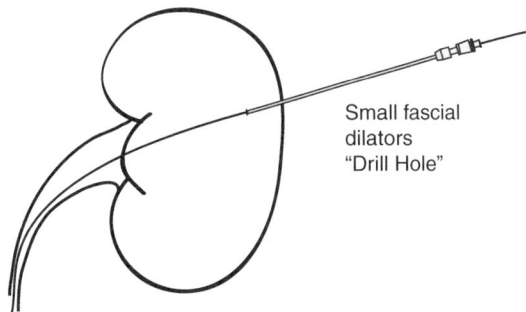

Fig. 13 Initial dilation of the kidney parenchyma with fine fascial dilators

Next, fascial dilators are passed over the wire, to create a rounded nephrostomy track of 12 French. This track is small, the dilators literally "drilling" the circular track (Fig. 13).

Following this, a "long grey" internal stent is passed over the guide wire. This "long grey" is long and may be unwieldy. It requires the surgeon to hold the operative hands wide apart. In some collecting systems where there is only a small space, only a small length of the leading edge is inside the collecting system, in which case the wire can be easily displaced during external manipulations of the "long grey" and Amplatz dilators.

The Amplatz dilators are exchanged serially over the "long grey". Each dilator is removed and upsized seriatim. Most tracks are dilated to 24- or 26-French size. The large dilators separate rather than "drill" the parenchyma to produce a stellate "split", rather like an open surgical nephrotomy.

They do not "drill" like the smaller fascial dilators. As these larger dilators separate rather than cut the parenchyma, they do not damage the parenchyma or renal vessels (Fig. 14).

Balloon Dilators

Note the complexity of the equipment.

Fig. 14 Subsequent upsizing of the nephrostomy track with larger dilators

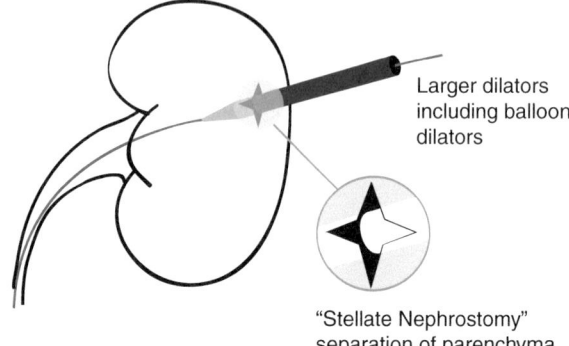

The balloon dilatation procedure involves a standard needle puncture, fascial dilators, a pump and pressure gauge, a balloon device and Amplatz sheath (Fig. 15).

Some balloon systems also incorporate a large Amplatz dilator.

Note that the inflated balloon tapers towards its tip. This may cause balloon extrusion if there is not a sufficient portion of the shaft of the balloon within the collecting system (Fig. 16).

The pump is disposable. Balloon track dilatation is monitored by II to confirm uniform dilatation of the balloon along the track. A standard Amplatz sheath is then passed over the balloon directly or, in some devices, over an Amplatz dilator.

Car Aerial

This system is reusable and can be resterilised (being metal).

The inner rod is long and rigid and can be cumbersome.

The car aerial dilators have a very snug fit (Fig. 17).

The flat distal end may push the kidney away.

Successive dilators fit snugly over the preceding dilator.

Occasionally the leading end can be difficult to pass through rigid tissues such as scar.

Many users of car aerial dilators switch to the serial Amplatz dilators in this scenario.

Single-Stage Dilator (Webb)

This it is a simple and cheap system. It comprises only one dilator and an Amplatz sheath.

The tip is tapered, sharp at the point, fits snugly over a guide wire and is polished or teflon coated so that it is slippery and passes easily through tissues (Fig. 18).

Appendix II: PCNL Workshop

Fig. 15 The components of a balloon dilation set

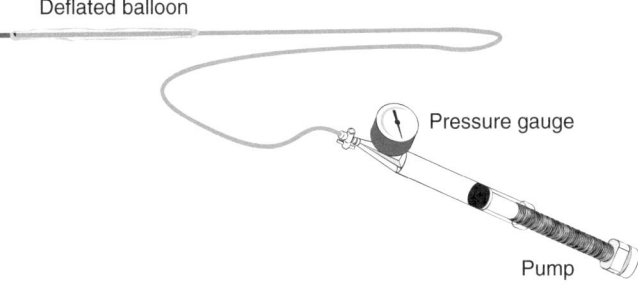

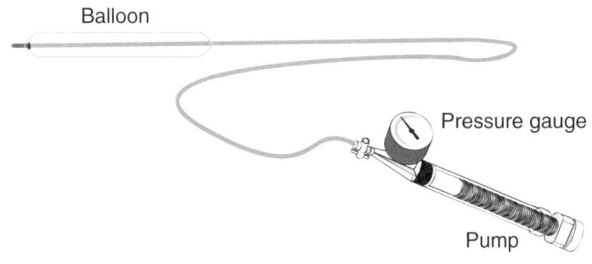

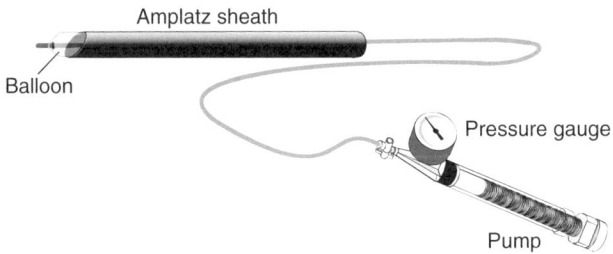

There is a line on the proximal shaft of the dilator. This is a safety marker. When the base of the Amplatz sheath is at that mark, the tip of the Amplatz sheath is at but not beyond the shoulder of the dilator. This allows the surgeon to safely insert the Amplatz sheath without imaging.

Amplatz Sheath

This tube provides a nephrocutaneous conduit which can be introduced over all varieties of renal dilators (Fig. 19).

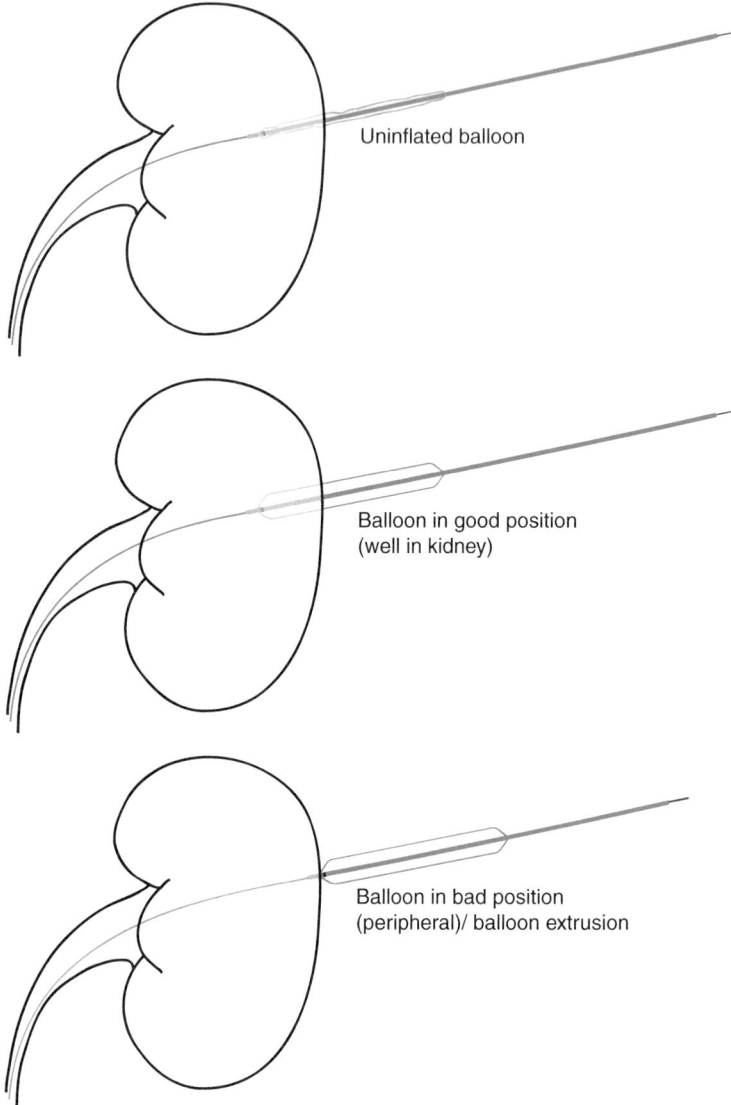

Fig. 16 Balloon dilation of the kidney and balloon extrusion

Note that the proximal end of the sheath is perpendicular to the shaft and round, whereas distally the opening is angulated and oval. The leading edge is bevelled and sharp. Rotating the sheath with insertion allows it to slide easily over the dilator and through the body wall layers.

Note that a 24-French dilator has an external circumference of 24 mm and that the accompanying Amplatz sheath is almost identical internally.

Appendix II: PCNL Workshop

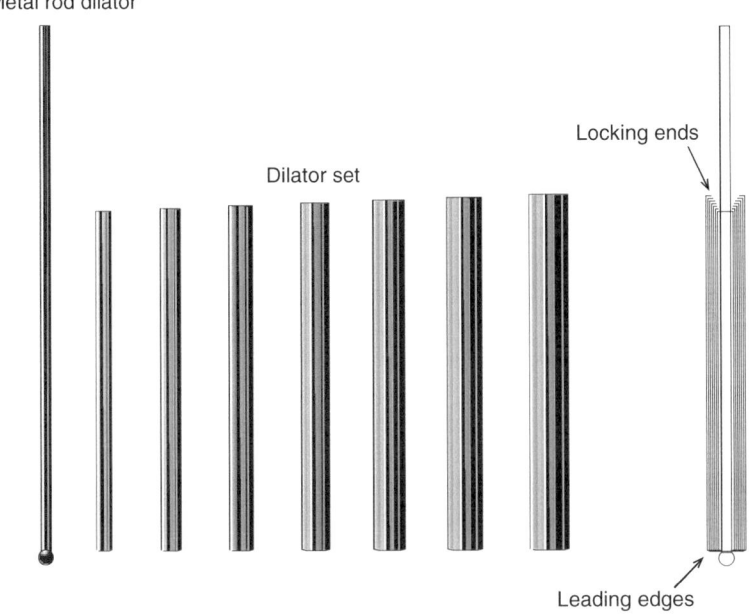

Fig. 17 Alken metal dilator

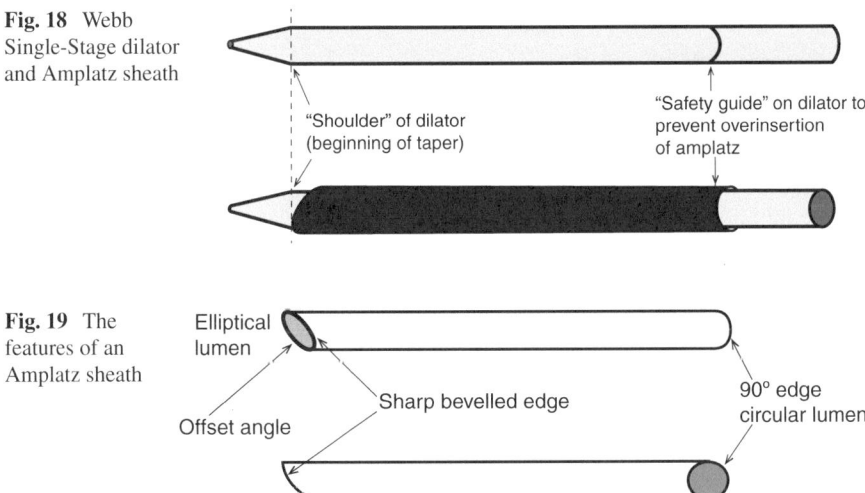

Fig. 18 Webb Single-Stage dilator and Amplatz sheath

Fig. 19 The features of an Amplatz sheath

By cutting an Amplatz sheath with scissors on opposite sides, the ends can be separated to provide a "short sheath" and also give the option to "peel away" the Amplatz sheath after insertion of a nephrostomy.

Tasks

Guide Wires

Examine the variety of guide wires.

Look at the tips, straight, "floppy" or "J" shaped.

Feed the tip of the "J-wire" into the "Golf T" introducer. Note how the wire is straightened by the introducer. Introduce the "J-wire" into the nephrostomy needle sheath using the "Golf T" introducer.

Look at the proximal (non-leading) end of the guide wire. Note that it is stiff and sharp (and so potentially traumatic).

Bend the guide wires to coil and kink them. Note that metallic coiled wires will kink and cannot be straightened. You cannot insert a dilator past a kink.

Slippery wires will not kink. However, they are springy and can "flick out" once kinked and can be easily displaced at surgery if not secured and held.

Wet the hydrophilic guide wires.

Holding the wires between two hands, pull the hands apart and note how the hands slip on the guide wire and cannot grip it.

Take an artery forceps and crush the jaws onto the hydrophilic and metallic guide wires directly. This trauma to the metallic guide wire renders it useless, but the hydrophilic wires are resistant to damage.

PCN Puncture Needles

Examine the puncture needles.

Remove the sheath from the needle.

Note the bevelled leading tip of the needle sheath.

Replace the sheath onto the needle.

Puncture a kidney (slowly) from the convex surface. Note that the tip of the needle initially indents the capsule and then perforates the capsule and kidney with a distinct "give". This can be felt during surgery (Fig. 20).

Dilator Systems

Use each of the four systems for renal dilatation.

To create a track into a calyx, pass the stiff or proximal end of a hydrophilic guide wire upwards along the ureter and through the renal pelvis to exit through the renal capsule (Fig. 21).

Use this guide wire for dilation with each type of dilator system.

Commence with the Amplatz dilatation system.

Note the "drilling" effect of the initial 8- and 10-Fr fascial dilators (Fig. 22).

Note that as the size of the dilators is increased, the nephrostomy begins to split and separate creating a "stellate" nephrotomy (Fig. 23).

Appendix II: PCNL Workshop

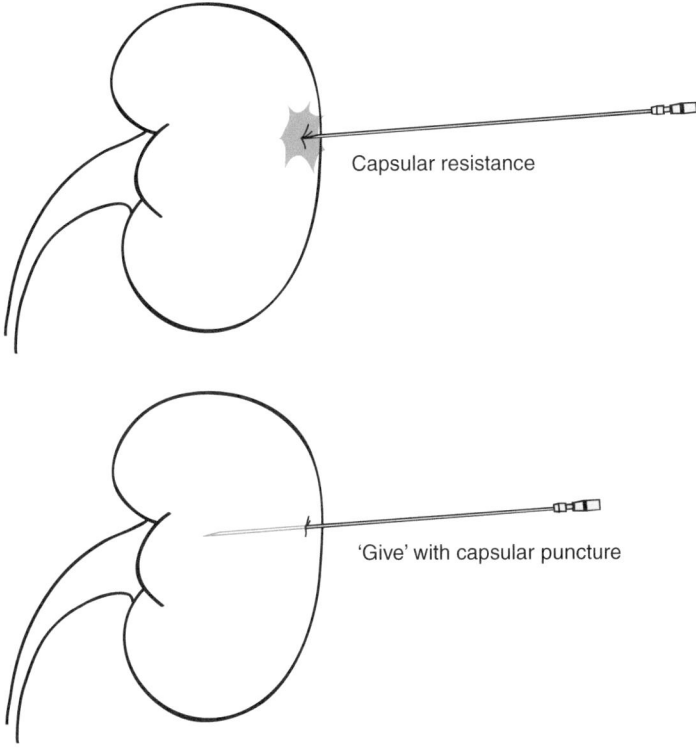

Fig. 20 The "sensation" of the initial needle puncture of the kidney

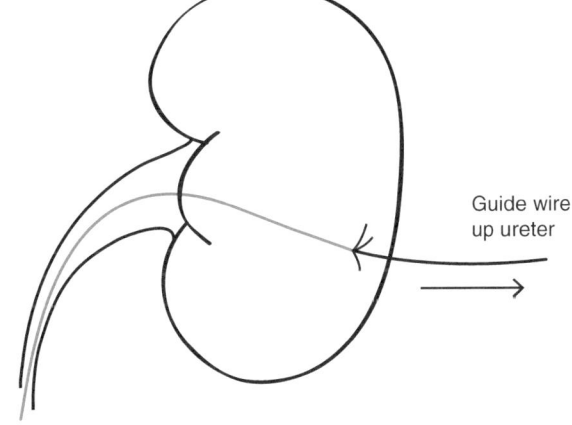

Fig. 21 To simulate a puncture, a guide wire is first pushed through the kidney in a retrograde fashion

Note that apart from separating the parenchyma, the larger dilators do not damage the kidney.

Once the final dilator is placed within the kidney, insert an Amplatz sheath, rotating it over the dilator until it is well within the collecting system. Leave the guide wire in situ.

Fig. 22 First pass small fascial dilators over the guide wire

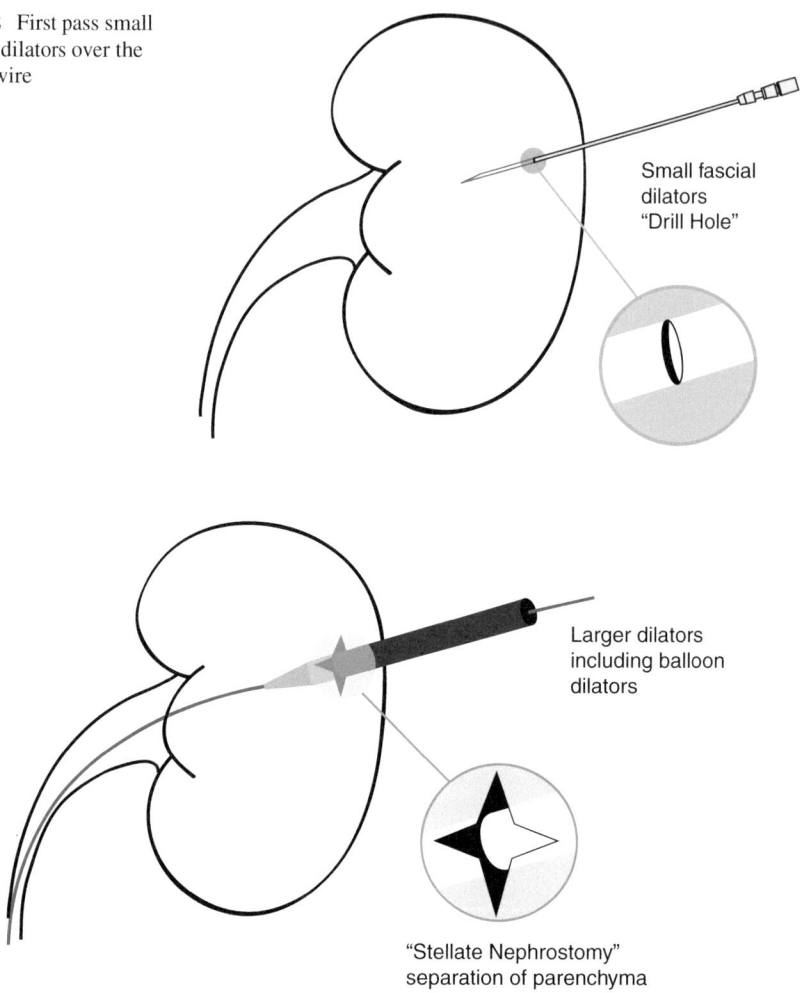

Fig. 23 Then pass larger dilators over the guide wire

Balloon Dilatation

Repeat the above.

Note that it is a multistage procedure. Note that the balloon needs to be well within the collecting system to be stable, and that if the tapered tip of the balloon is not well within the kidney, inflation may result in balloon extrusion (Fig. 24).

Again, place the Amplatz dilator over the final balloon or dilator (varies from maker to maker). Observe that the track created using balloon dilation is identical to that made by serial dilators.

Appendix II: PCNL Workshop

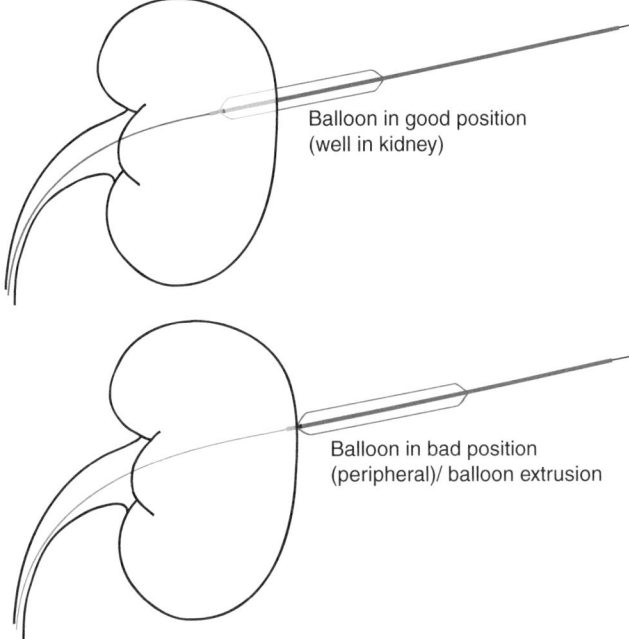

Fig. 24 Insert the deflated balloon well inside the kidney and inflate. Do the same with the balloon at the outer edge of the kidney

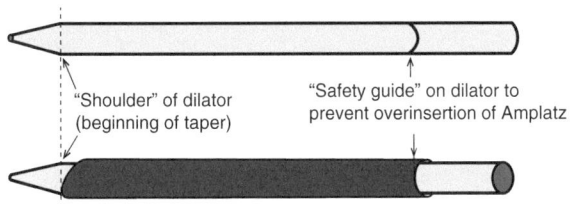

Fig. 25 Observe that the Webb SSD has a proximal marker so the surgeon can avoid over advancement of the Amplatz sheath

Single-Stage Dilator

Feel the tip of the dilator. Note that it is sharp, tapered and slippery (either from polishing or a hydrophilic coating).

Note that the tip fits snugly over the guide wire.

Note the Amplatz safety marker proximally on the shaft (Fig. 25). Pass the single-stage dilator over the guide wire, rotating it into the kidney (Fig. 26).

Note the simplicity and speed of the dilatation.

Perform the dilator introduction slowly. Watch how the tip of the dilator initially mimics the small fascial dilators from the Amplatz system by "drilling" a hole. As the dilator is introduced further, the parenchyma separates to create an atraumatic nephrotomy, similar to the serial and balloon dilator systems.

Pass an Amplatz sheath over the dilator up to the proximal safety marker (Fig. 27).

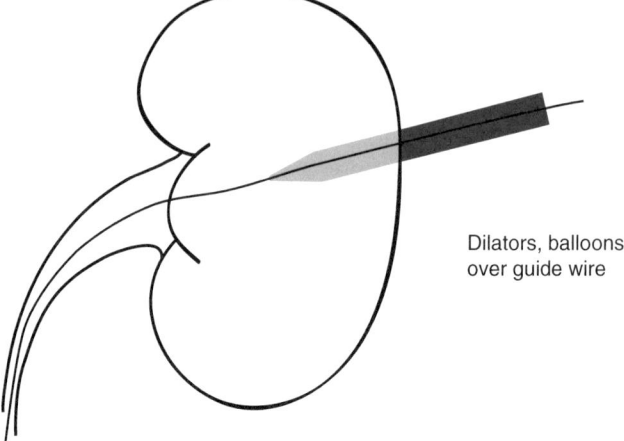

Fig. 26 Insert the SSD dilator and then introduce the Amplatz sheath over the dilator

Dilators, balloons over guide wire

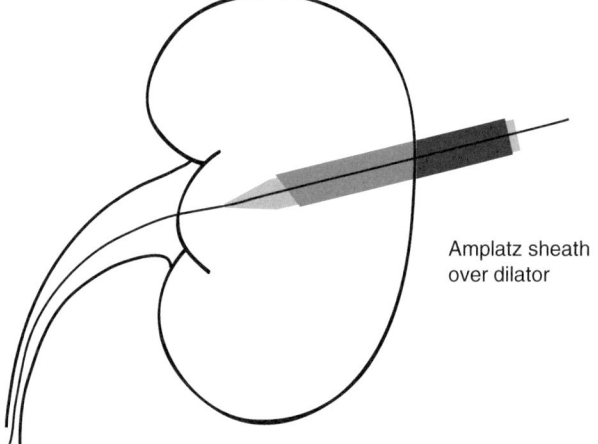

Fig. 27 Rotate and advance the Amplatz sheath until its proximal end is at the circular safety marker on the dilator

Amplatz sheath over dilator

Car Aerial

Pass the internal rod over the guide wire. Then, pass the metal dilators seriatim over the rod.

At the end of the dilatation, an Amplatz sheath is passed over the final car aerial dilator.

In some car aerial systems, the final "dilator" is the nephroscope sheath. This system is "closed" and requires continuous flow irrigation.

Fig. 28 Examine the features of the Cope loop nephrostomy

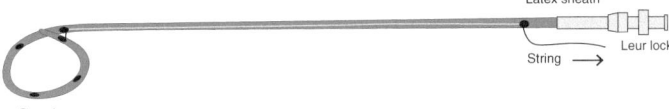

Fig. 29 Remove the dilator and insert a Cope nephrostomy into the kidney

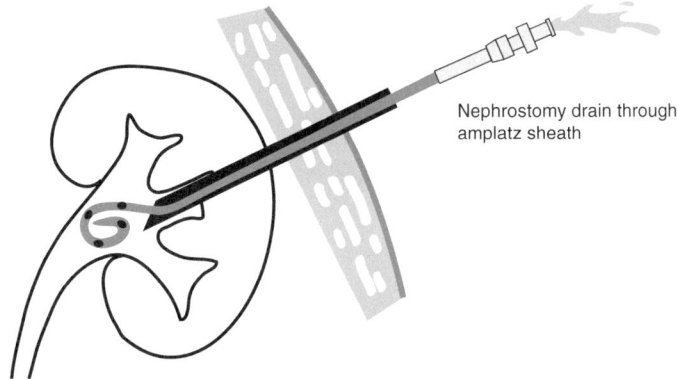

Nephrostomy

Inspect the Cope loop nephrostomy.

Note the string from the tip of the nephrostomy lumen re-entering a few centimetres proximally to the loop. This string fixes the retaining loop when it is pulled proximally. Note that the string exits at the proximal end of the nephrostomy tubing through a small hole. This opening may leak contrast or urine, so it must be covered with a rubber sheath. The sheath closes the hole and fixes the string, which in turn maintains the retaining loop in the renal pelvis (Fig. 28).

Note that the Cope nephrostomy loop has a "memory". This can be used to advantage when placing the nephrostomy.

Pull the drawstring to close the retaining loop and secure the drawstring proximally by rolling the rubber sheath down. Place a finger in the Cope loop. You will observe that the loop is firmly retained by the string.

It is important to realise that this drawstring must be fully released by rolling back the latex sheath before removal of a Cope nephrostomy. Otherwise significant renal trauma can be inflicted by forcibly extracting a closed loop.

Straighten the Cope loop over a guide wire in one of your dilator specimens in which you have placed an Amplatz sheath. Advance the Cope loop to the inside of the kidney over the guide wire, remove the guide wire, tighten the string and fix (Fig. 29).

The "peel away" technique of Amplatz sheath removal.

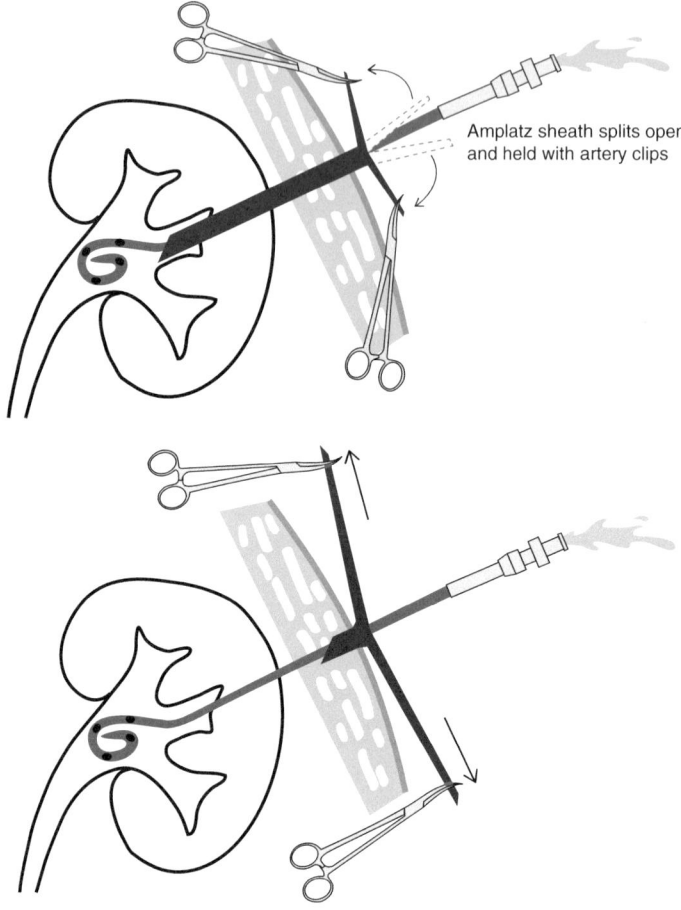

Fig. 30 Divide the outer Amplatz sheath in either side vertically for 2 cm with heavy scissors to create "flaps". Grasp each flap with an artery forcep and pull apart to split and extrude the sheath around the nephrostomy

Using scissors cut the Amplatz sheath on either side (i.e. 0° and 180°). Peel away to split the Amplatz in two and leave the nephrostomy and the kidney (Figs. 30 and 31).

Station 3: Techniques for Difficult Renal Punctures and Renal Access

Equipment Required

1. Kidneys – two per group
2. Hydrophilic guide wire

Appendix II: PCNL Workshop

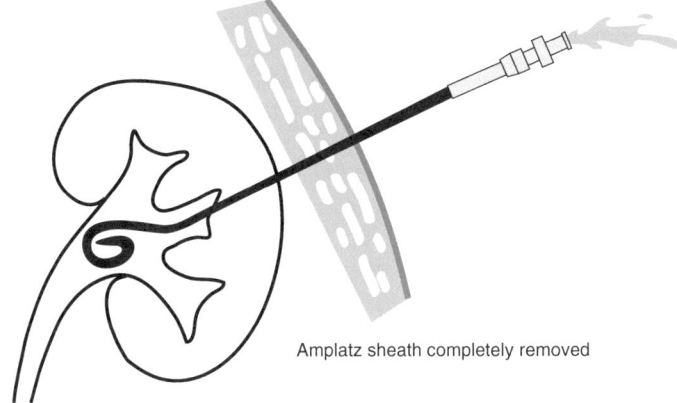

Fig. 31 Note how the nephrostomy is undisturbed by this manouvre

Amplatz sheath completely removed

3. Two artery forceps
4. Serial dilators or Webb dilators
5. Large knife and scalpel
6. Puncture needle and sheath.
7. Alligator forceps only if available to be used in the porcine model

Aims

To learn a number of options for gaining renal access in complex or difficult scenarios such as large staghorn calculi, calculi that completely occupy a calyx and calculi in calyceal diverticulum and for access to a "parallel lie" stone.

To learn the technique of creating a nephrostomy track through the renal parenchyma by separating the renal parenchyma under vision using alligator grasping forceps. (Artery forceps are used for the workshop.)

To learn the method of creating a "UGW":

Observe that a UGW fixed proximally and distally by artery forceps provides a stable means of renal access that cannot be displaced, aligns the kidney and the dilatation track and provides a stable guide wire for dilatation without the kidney flipping or rotating.

To understand the theory of the "Y" puncture, note that the shaft of the "Y" is the portion of the track from the renal capsule to the skin. The "V" of the "Y" is formed by the two punctures through the renal substance into neighbouring calyces.

Note that this technique is suited to calyces that are close, usually "parallel lie" calyces, and not calyces that are widely separated. Only a short second puncture track can be created using a "Y" puncture.

The usual clinical scenario is between an anterior and posterior calyx.

Creating a UGW through the initial puncture is the first stage of the "Y" puncture. The UGW provides a stable track for subsequent dilatation and helps stabilise

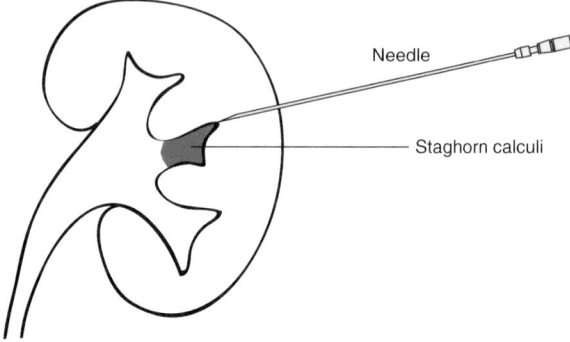

Fig. 32 An example of a calyx that does not have enough space to enable placement of a stable guide wire

the kidney during the creation of the second creation of the line of the "Y" into the neighbouring calyx.

The "Y puncture" technique can be used "electively", e.g. to gain access to a polar calyceal diverticulum.

This approach is particularly useful for polar punctures, where the kidney is very mobile.

Situations in which a guide wire cannot be placed in a stable fashion into the collecting system:

In scenarios such as a complete staghorn calculus, a stone firmly impacted into a non-dilated calyx or calculi in a calyceal diverticulum, it may not be possible to introduce a sufficient length of guide wire within the collecting system that is stable enough for track dilatation (Fig. 32).

This exercise describes the technique of creating a "stable" guide wire by coiling a length of wire in the retroperitoneum outside the kidney.

This gives the guide wire enough stability for a track to be dilated directly onto the stone. Then the surgeon can "excavate" the stone with a sonotrode, creating space between the stone and collecting system, thereby allowing the surgeon to pass a guide wire under vision into the renal pelvis and ureter between the stone and the calyceal wall.

Note that the alligator forceps have a blunt rounded tip. They are not sharp or traumatic.

These can be inserted under vision into the outer renal parenchyma alongside a guide wire and opened, thereby creating a nephrostomy track mechanically. This technique separates rather than cuts parenchyma (similar to an open nephrotomy), so it is atraumatic.

This endoscopic nephrostomy technique is very useful when a calculus is very impacted and the surgeon cannot safely advance a dilator into the kidney.

Tasks

Universal Guide Wire

Take a kidney and pass the stiff end of the guide wire up the ureter to perforate the kidney (Fig. 33).

Appendix II: PCNL Workshop

Fig. 33 Insert a guide wire retrograde from the ureter through the kidney

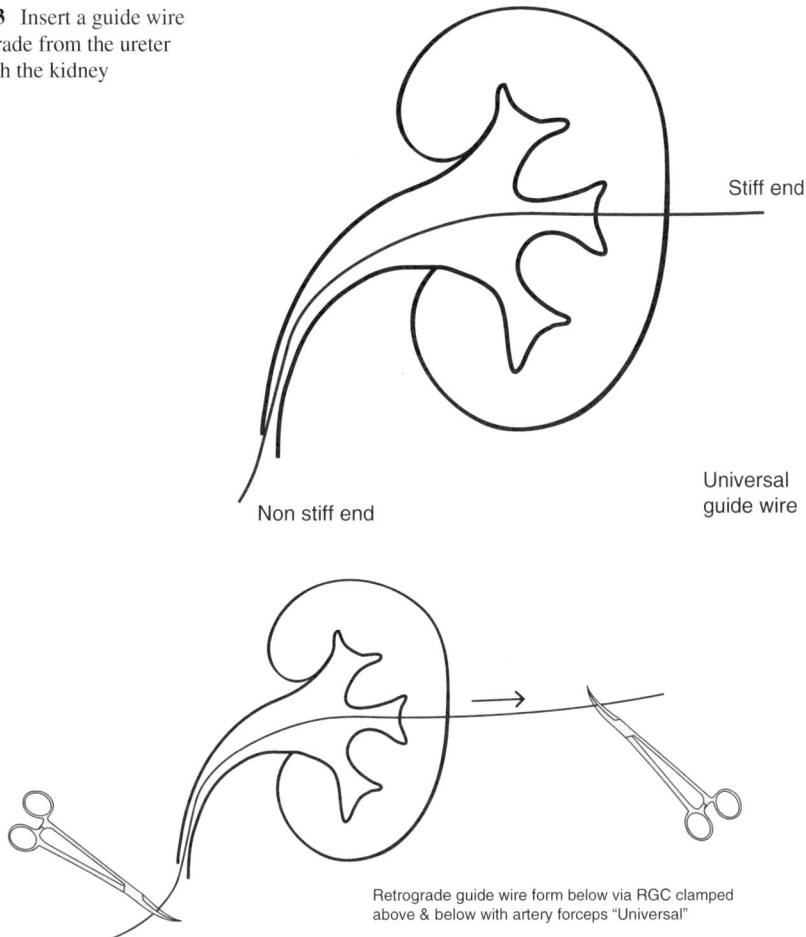

Fig. 34 Grasp and fix either end of the guide wire with artery forceps to create a UGW

Grasp each end of the guide wire to mimic a "universal guide wire" (Fig. 34). Put tension on the forceps and note that kidney aligns along the guide wire.

"Y" Puncture

Pass a dilator (a single stage is easiest for this procedure) over a guide wire into the kidney (Fig. 35).

Bivalve the kidney horizontally along the dilator leaving the guide wire in situ (Fig. 36).

Pass a needle from the capsular entry point of the dilator into a neighbouring calyx. Through that guide wire sheath introduce a second guide wire into the neighbouring calyx (Fig. 37).

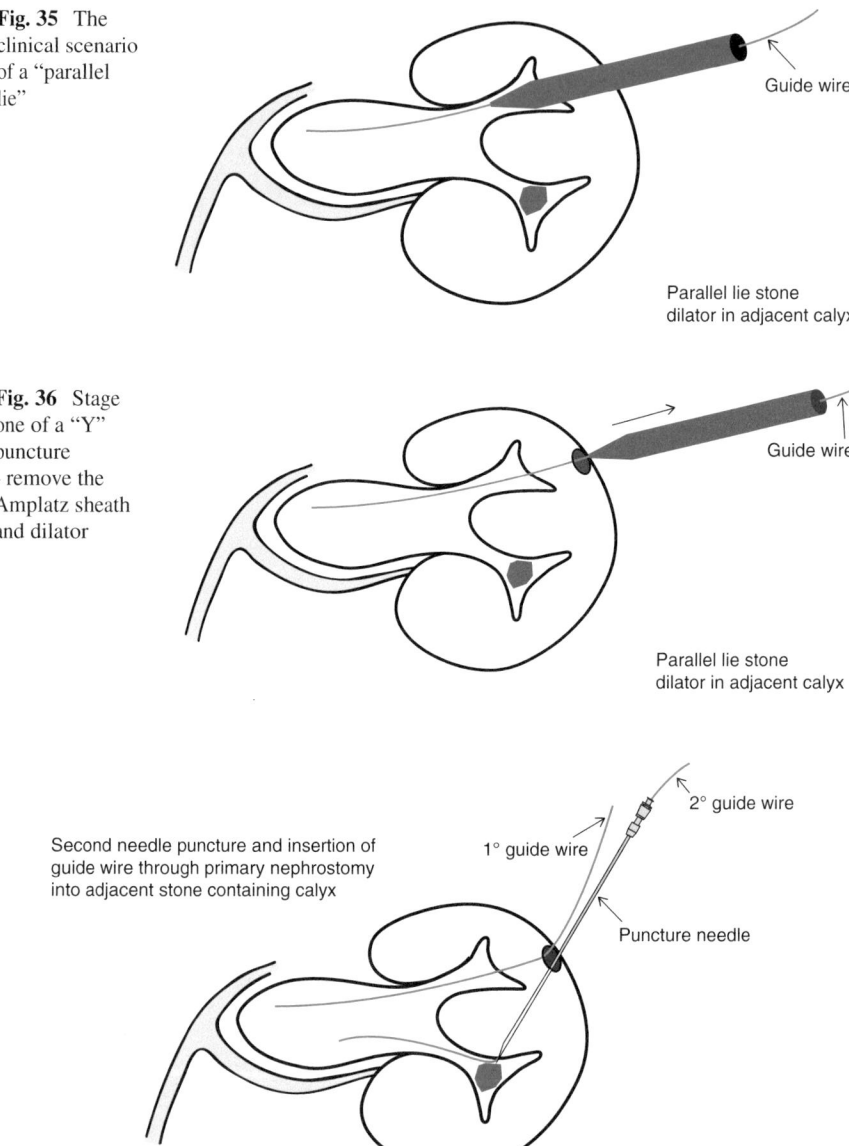

Fig. 35 The clinical scenario of a "parallel lie"

Fig. 36 Stage one of a "Y" puncture - remove the Amplatz sheath and dilator

Fig. 37 Stage two - puncture into the adjacent calyx through the primary entry portal

Remove the original dilator from its calyx; pass it over the second guide wire entering through the same outer border entry portal of the primary nephrostomy. Pass the dilator on the second guide wire into the adjacent calyx to create the "Y" puncture (Fig. 38).

Appendix II: PCNL Workshop

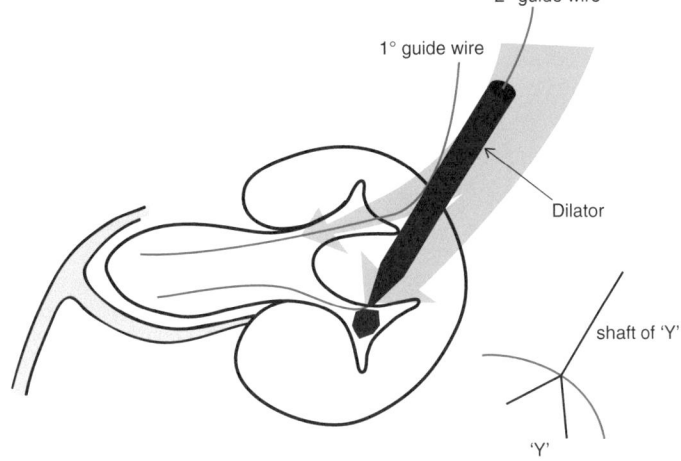

Fig. 38 Stage three - insert a guide wire and then a dilator and sheath into the adjacent calyx

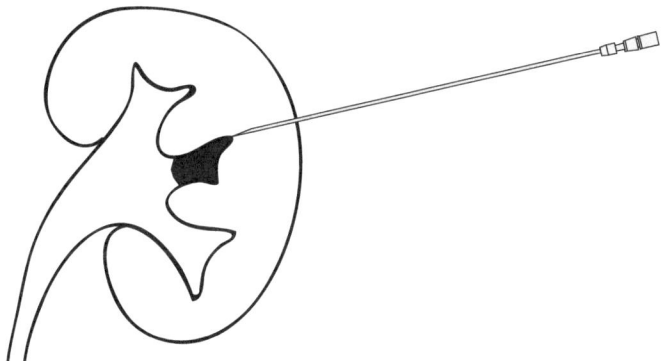

Fig. 39 The retroperitoneal guide wire (RPGW) technique for when there is no space around the stone to place a guide wire

Creating a Track When One Is Unable to Establish a Guide Wire in the Collecting System (Fig. 39)

Take the kidney in one hand and a nephrostomy needle in the other

Pass the needle through the kidney to the other side (Fig. 40), remove the needle, leave the transparent sheath and pass the floppy end of a guide wire through the kidney to simulate the retroperitoneal coil (Fig. 41). Dilate over the guide wire with a single-stage dilator and introduce an Amplatz sheath (Fig. 42).

Endoscopic Nephrotomy

Take the kidney and pass the guide wire retrograde to form a universal guide wire (Fig. 43).

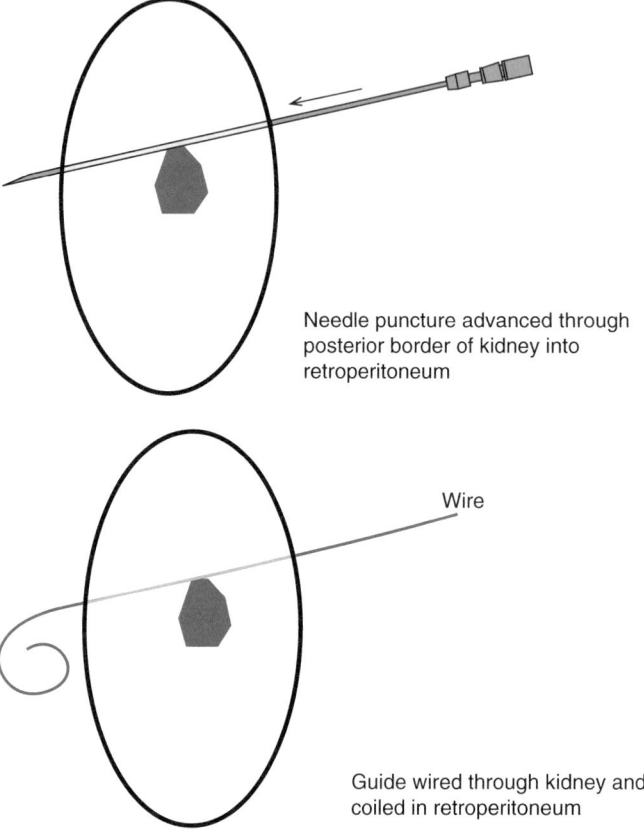

Fig. 40 Kidney lateral view - pass the needle and sheath through the kidney to exit posteriorly and remove the needle

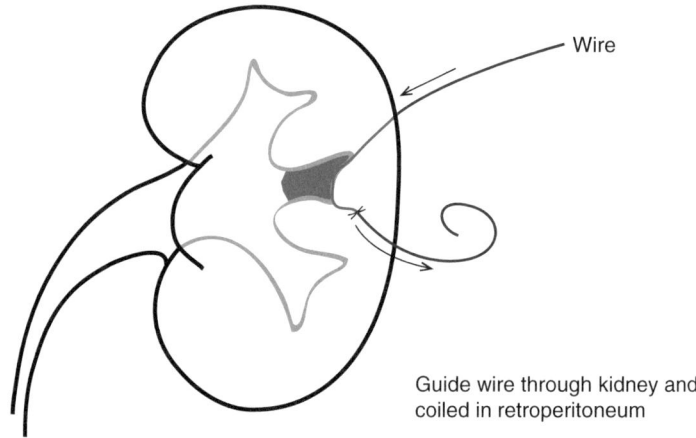

Fig. 41 Kidney anterior view - thread sufficient guide wire through the kidney to make it stable

Appendix II: PCNL Workshop 223

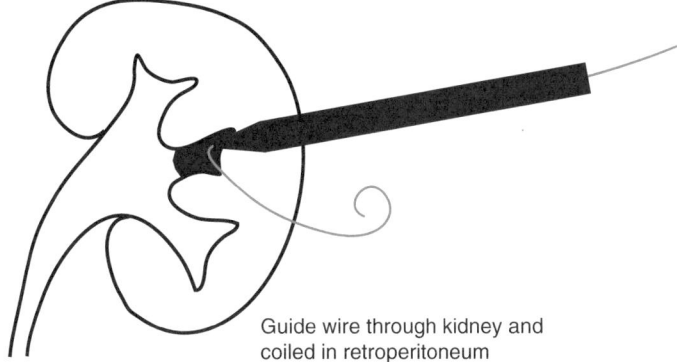

Fig. 42 Insert a dilator over the guide wire into the kidney

Guide wire through kidney and coiled in retroperitoneum

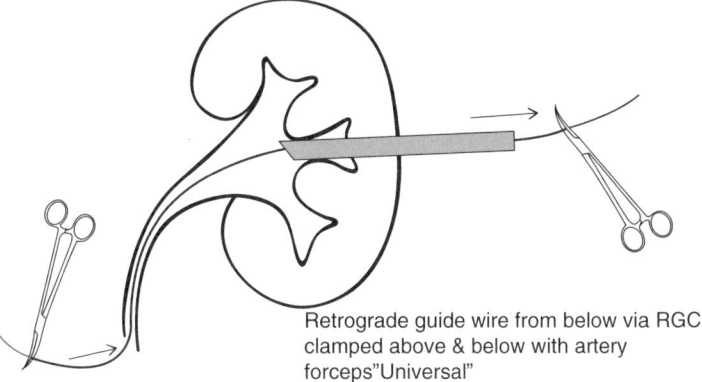

Fig. 43 Pass an Amplatz sheath, remove the dilator and fix the wire with artery forceps

Retrograde guide wire from below via RGC clamped above & below with artery forceps"Universal"

If available, use alligator forceps (but if not, use artery forceps). Gently place the tips of the forceps alongside the guide wire into the parenchyma (Fig. 44).

Gently open the jaws to create an atraumatic nephrostomy (Fig. 45).

Station 4: Trauma to the Kidney, Renal Vessels and Collecting System during PCNL

Equipment Required

Kidneys – two per group
    Hydrophilic guide wires
    Amplatz sheaths
    Dilators (Amplatz, serial, balloon, single stage)
    Large sharp knife or scalpel

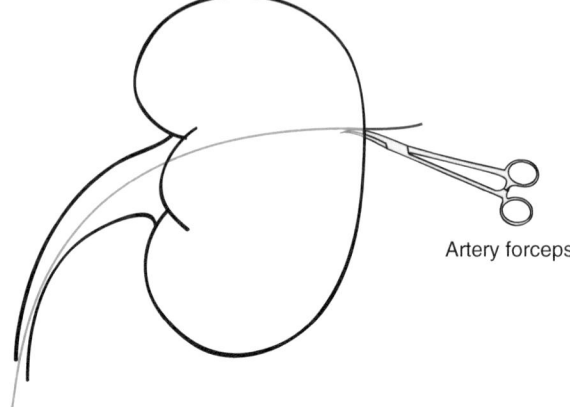

Fig. 44 Remove the Amplatz sheath and insert the tips of an artery forcep alongside the guide wire to simulate Alligator forceps through a nephroscope

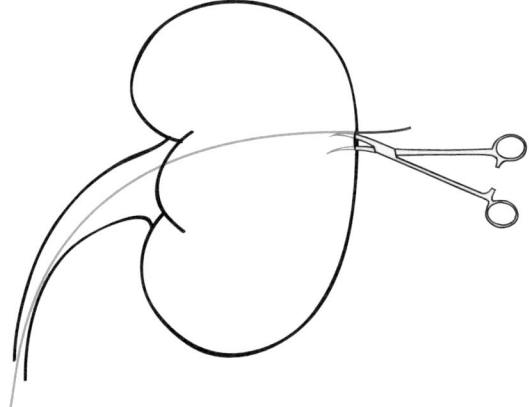

Fig. 45 Gently separate the tips to create an atraumatic nephrotomy as you can do under vision with Alligator forceps through a nephroscope

Aims

To demonstrate that a safe puncture entering the tip of the calyx affords maximal intrarenal access with the least trauma.

To demonstrate that the leading end of the Amplatz sheath can cause severe parenchymal, vascular and collecting system damage if not inserted correctly over a dilator.

To demonstrate that a renal puncture that is too medial is likely to cause significant vascular, parenchymal and collecting system damage and compromise intrarenal endoscopic access.

Appendix II: PCNL Workshop

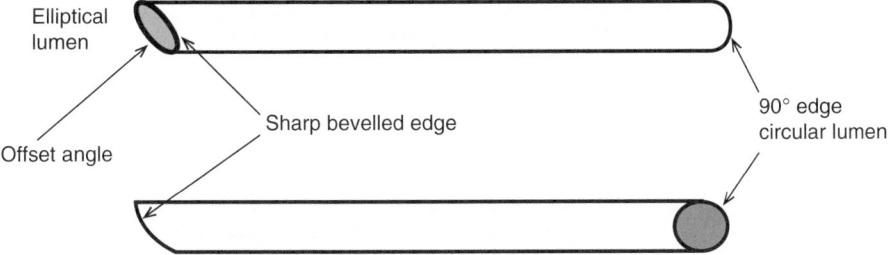

Fig. 46 The Amplatz sheath has a bevelled oval advancing end and a round outer end both of which are sharp

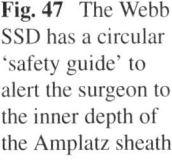

Fig. 47 The Webb SSD has a circular 'safety guide' to alert the surgeon to the inner depth of the Amplatz sheath

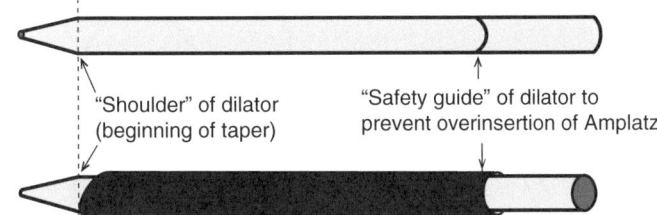

Observations

Amplatz Sheath

Examine an Amplatz sheath. Note that the leading edge is sharp and has the ability to cut and core (Fig. 46).

You will observe that if the Amplatz is "over-advanced", in other words, past the shoulder (Fig. 47) of the dilator, the leading sharp edge can cut the parenchyma and collecting system.

Dilators

A safe track is one that enters the tip of the calyx, thereby traversing the least amount of parenchyma. In doing so it enters the calyx where the collecting system attached to the parenchyma and so is resistant to displacement or tearing (Fig. 48).

By entering the calyx at its tip as the dilator progresses medially, it is safely separated from the large vessels in the renal sinus by the collecting system.

By entering the kidney through the thinnest amount of parenchyma, movement of instruments is over a narrow fulcrum allowing maximum excursion of the tip of instrument, with the least amount of parenchymal trauma (Fig. 49).

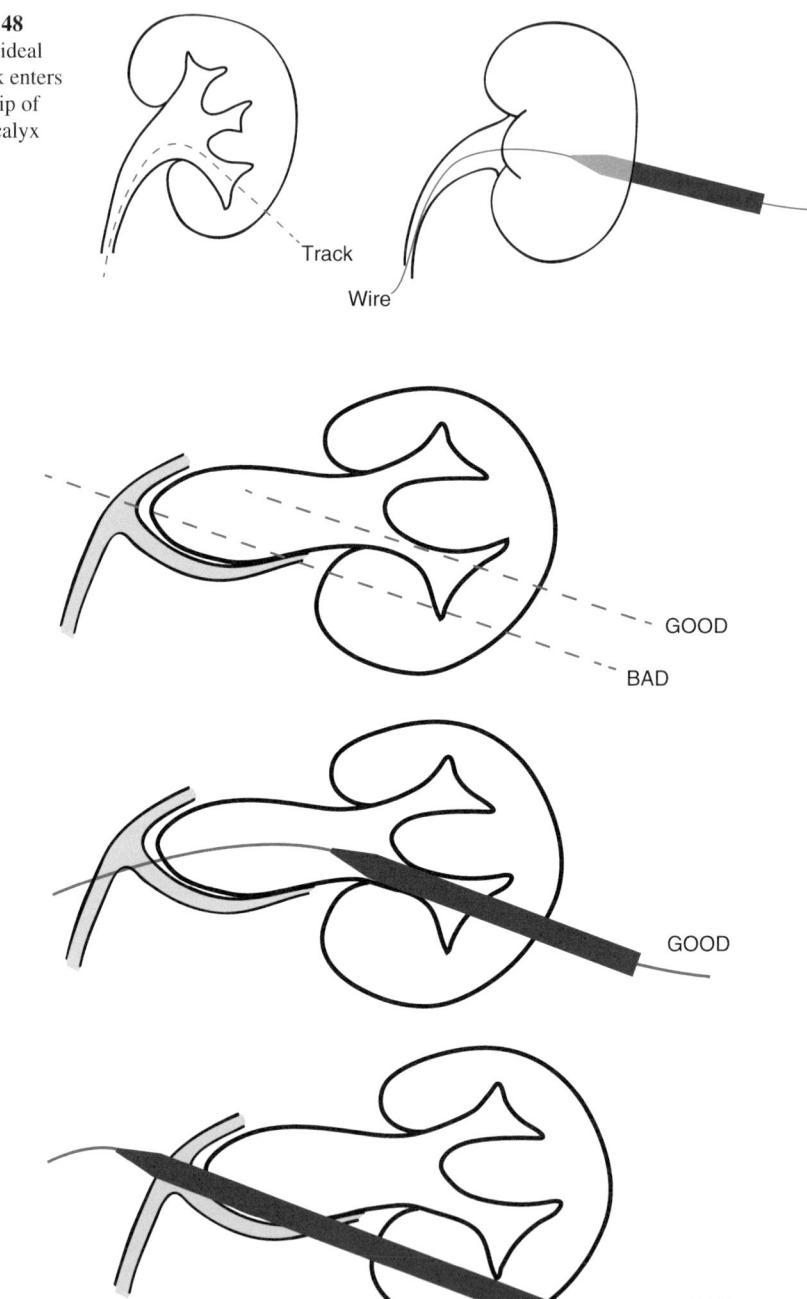

Fig. 48 The ideal track enters the tip of the calyx

Fig. 49 Examples of good and traumatic nephrostomy tracks

Fig. 50 Poor needle track

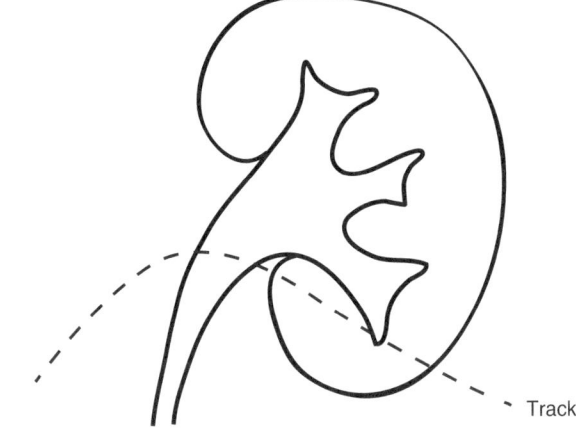

Fig. 51 Damage from dilation over a badly placed guide wire

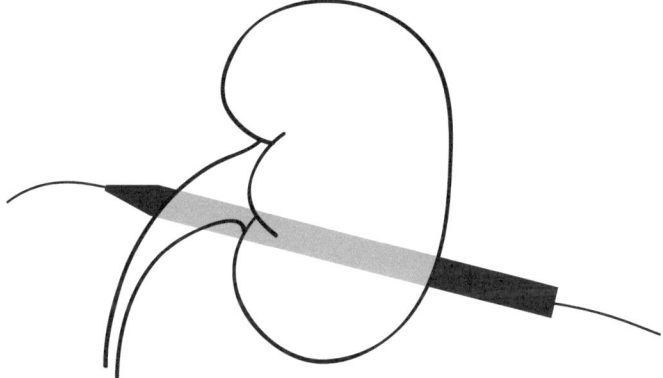

Nephrostomy Track: Bad Track

A bad track is the opposite of a good track! When a dilator enters the kidney medially, it punctures the proximal infundibulum or the pelvis and transverses a large segment of parenchyma (Fig. 50).

As this track traverses the renal sinus, instruments are in direct contact with the segmental vessels (Fig. 51).

If the track enters the infundibulum or pelvis where it is unsupported, it can tear the collecting system resulting in extravasation of contrast, blood, irrigation fluid and stone fragments.

A long parenchymal traverse results in a long parenchyma results in "fulcrum". This significantly limits intrarenal mobility and access. Manipulation of the nephroscope through a long parenchyma track causes extensive splitting and trauma to the parenchyma and collecting system (see Fig. 49).

Tasks

Amplatz Trauma

(a) Parenchymal trauma

Take a kidney and an Amplatz sheath without a dilator.

Screw the Amplatz into the kidney to take a sharp core of parenchyma (Fig. 52).

This is the trauma caused when the Amplatz sheath is advanced beyond the leading shoulder of the tip of the dilator (e.g. when the dilator shaft is not fully within the collecting system) (Fig. 53).

Establish a universal guide wire as previously described.

Place the dilator over the guide wire with the shoulder approximately one centimetre through the parenchyma.

Over-advance the Amplatz sheath over the latter so that it is at least 1–1.5 cm distal to the shoulder of the dilator (Fig. 54).

Divide the kidney over the sheath and observe the trauma to the infundibulum (Fig. 55).

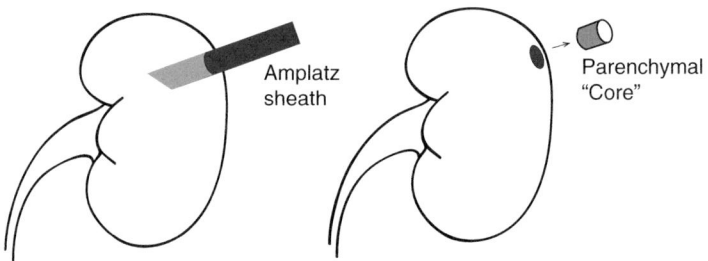

Fig. 52 "Amplatz Trauma" - parenchyma (without dilator)

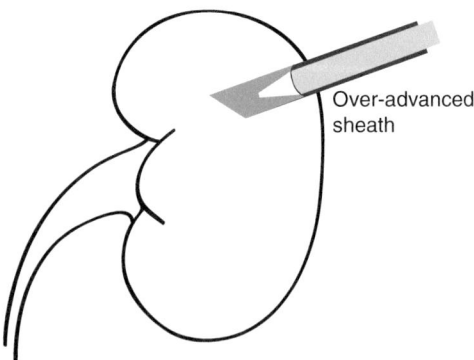

Fig. 53 "Amplatz Trauma" - parenchymal from over advancement of sheath over the dilator

Fig. 54 "Amplatz Trauma" - over advancement lacerating the calyceal neck

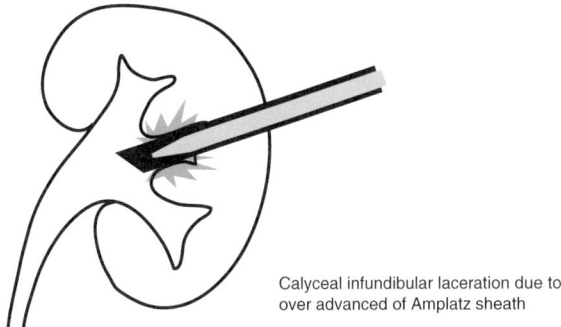

Calyceal infundibular laceration due to over advanced of Amplatz sheath

Fig. 55 "Amplatz Trauma" - lacerated calyx after removal of the sheath

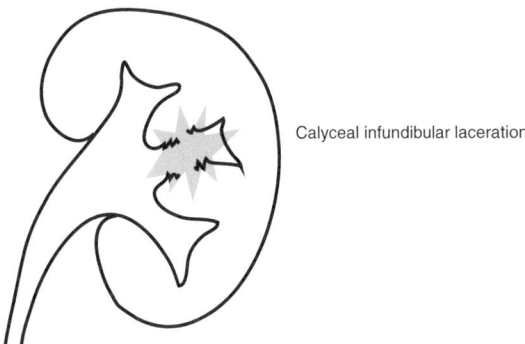

Calyceal infundibular laceration

Collecting System Trauma

Establishing a Good Track

Take a separate kidney, establish a universal guide wire, and pass a dilator to the renal pelvis.

Screw an Amplatz sheath over the dilator, so that the oval end is leading and distal to the dilator (Fig. 56).

Note that the Amplatz has the ability to lacerate the pelvic wall and amputate the pelvic ureteric junction (Fig. 57).

Take a kidney, establish a universal guide wire, pass the Amplatz dilator to the renal pelvis, and assess intrarenal mobility by angulating the dilator up and down (see Fig. 49).

Observe that there is minimal parenchymal damage.

Bivalve the kidney over the Amplatz and observe that the whole system, in other words the Amplatz sheath and therefore the nephroscope, is within the collecting system.

Examine the parenchymal track for trauma and splitting.

Fig. 56 "Amplatz Trauma" - inadvertent advancement of the sheath into the upper ureter lacerating the PUJ

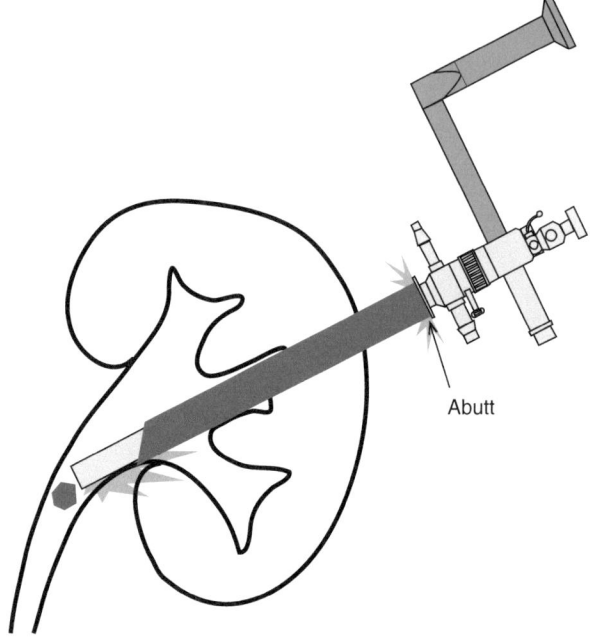

Over-advancement of the tip of the Amplatz sheath by the nephroscope unknowingly pushing the proximal end of Amplatz sheath

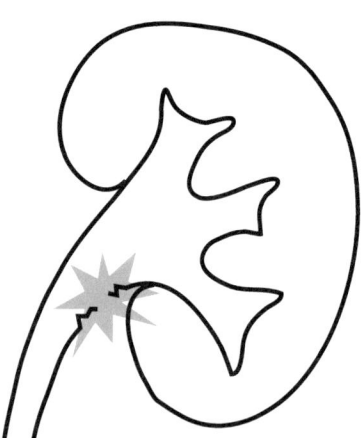

Fig. 57 The pelvis and ureter can be lacerated or even completely divided

Pelvis-PUJ laceration or dismembered

Appendix II: PCNL Workshop

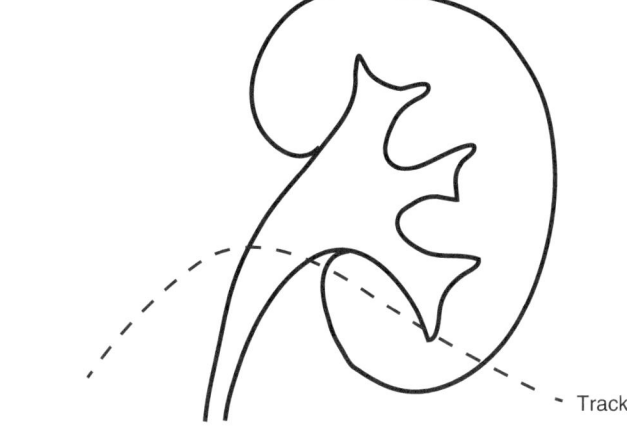

Fig. 58 Poor track puncture

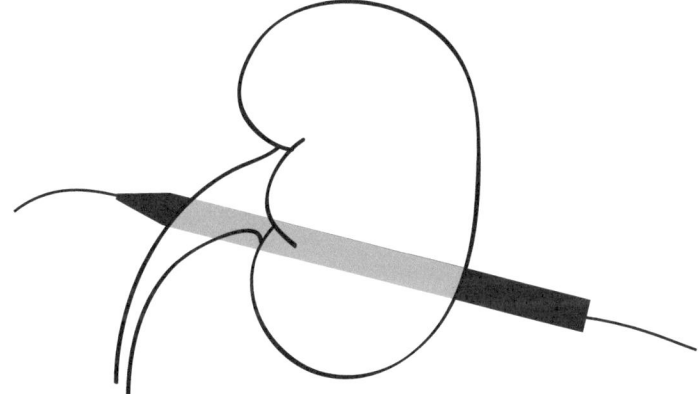

Fig. 59 Dilation of poor track puncture

Poor Track

Take a kidney and PCNL needle.

Puncture the kidney medially so that the needle traverses a long area of parenchyma, renal sinus and pelvis (Fig. 58).

Remove the needle, leave the external sheath, and insert a guide wire through the needle sheath.

Pass a dilator (a single stage is easiest) over the guide wire until it is into the pelvis or even through the other side of the pelvis (Fig. 59).

Pass an Amplatz over the guide wire.

Manipulate the dilator and Amplatz as previously described. Note how mobility is limited by the long intraparenchymal track. Observe that the manipulation of the dilator can result in tearing of the collecting system, splitting of the renal parenchyma and damage to the vessels within the renal sinus (see Fig. 49).

Station 5: Percutaneous Nephrolithotomy – Endoscopic Stone Fragmentation and Equipment

Equipment

Endoscopic tower, including light source camera and screen
    Ultrasonic and pneumatic lithotrite power sources
    Gas supply for the pneumatic lithotrite and saline irrigation and pump for the ultrasonic lithotrite
    Nephroscopes, either a rigid 30° or 90° crank handle varieties
    Flexible nephroscope (optional)
    Light cables
    Graspers – triradiate and alligator
    Ureteric baskets (varied)
    Stone dummies (chalk)
    Glass beaker in which to put the chalk and saline for nephroscopic fragmentation using in the sonotrode and pneumatic lithotrites
    Amplatz sheath
    Heavy scissors
    Two artery forceps

Aims

To familiarise the surgeon with the features of rigid nephroscopy, flexible nephroscopy, the various instruments available for stone extraction and the advantages and limitations and applications of endoscopic lithotrites.
    To appreciate the limitations and advantages of each instrument.
    To become familiar with ultrasonic and pneumatic stone fragmentation.
    To understand the relationship between the camera and endoscope orientation when using rigid and flexible endoscopes.

Observations

Note that the standard nephroscopes are rigid with straight working channels and "offset" lenses, either the 90° (crank handle) or 30° offset (Figs. 60 and 61).
    The offset lenses allows the passage of straight instruments such as pneumatic lithotrites, ultrasonic probes and rigid grasping forceps, as well as the flexible baskets, guide wires and laser fibres.
    Note that a cross section of most nephroscopes *is* usually oval rather than circular (Fig. 62).

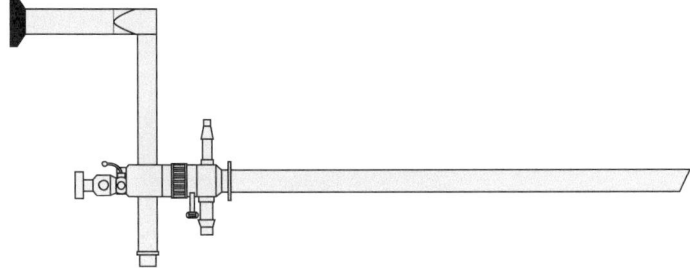

Fig. 60 Crank handle or 90° offset nephroscope

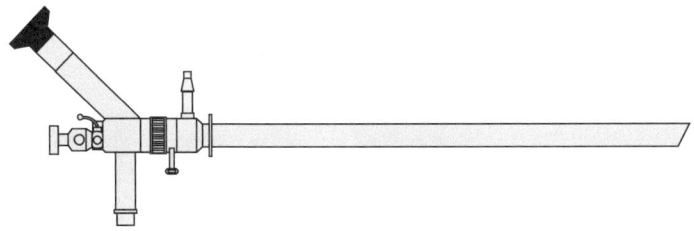

Fig. 61 Oblique or 30° offset nephroscope

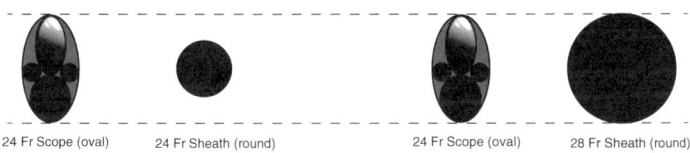

24 Fr Scope (oval)   24 Fr Sheath (round)   24 Fr Scope (oval)   28 Fr Sheath (round)

Fig. 62 Comparison of diameter and circumference

Therefore, the maximum diameter of an oval shaped nephroscope will be wider than the diameter of a circular Amplatz sheath of the same French gauge size.

Therefore, a nephroscope with a 24-French outer perimeter requires a 26 or 28 French.

Amplatz sheath (Fig. 63).

Observe that by holding the camera by the non-dominant hand and passing an instrument through the nephroscope, the instrument movement will appear as it rotates without disorientating the surgeon.

Note that there is a marker at six o'clock on the endoscopic image on the monitor that provides an extra orientation reference for the surgeon (Fig. 64).

By maintaining the camera in a fixed position, the location of this orientation marker remains static.

Note that the working end of the nephroscope is angled, so that during rotation, both the light and vision expand to provide a wider area of vision than a straight-ahead lens (Fig. 65).

Fig. 63 End view of 24 Fr Nephroscope in a 28 Fr Amplatz sheath

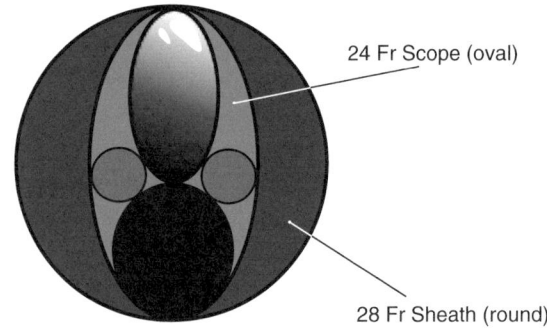

Fig. 64 Endoscopic view of the monitor with a 6 o'clock orientation marker on the screen

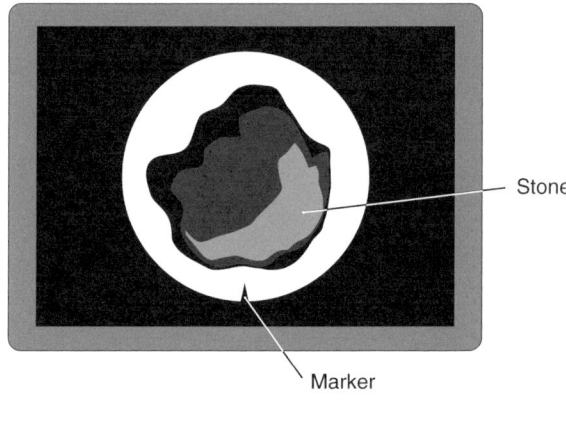

Fig. 65 Extended nephroscope view on rotation from the offset lens

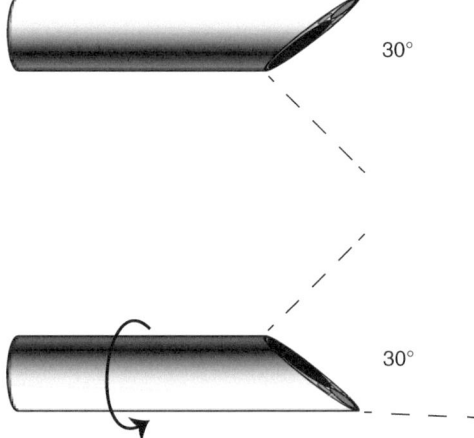

Appendix II: PCNL Workshop 235

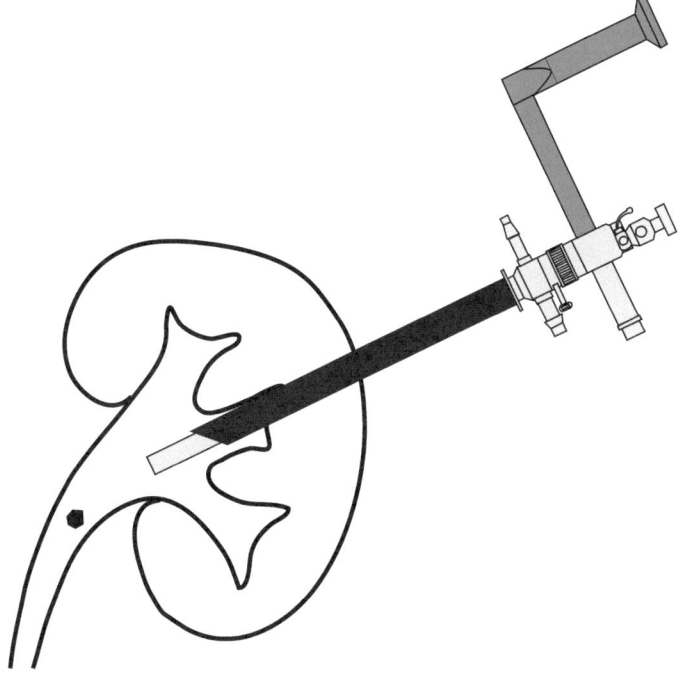

Fig. 66 The surgeon cannot see the inner leading edge of the Amplatz sheath when the nephroscope is fully inserted

Task

Place a nephroscope in an Amplatz sheath and note the limited excursion of the nephroscope above and below the ends of the Amplatz sheath.

Note the inability of the surgeon to see the inner end of an Amplatz sheath when the nephroscope is protruding from the sheath (Fig. 66).

Note that advancing the nephroscope while the Amplatz sheath is in contact with the nephroscope proximally "unconsciously" advances the Amplatz sheath forwards without the surgeon being aware (Fig. 67).

Examine the distal or operating end of a nephroscope and observe (Fig. 68).

1. Oval shape
2. Large instrument channel
3. Small irrigation channels
4. The light source
5. The angled lens and distribution of light

Place the nephroscope in a small Amplatz sheath and note that even though the French gauge is similar, the nephroscope may not be able to be introduced into the sheath itself or if it does fit, its excursion is compromised by friction between the nephroscope and the sheath.

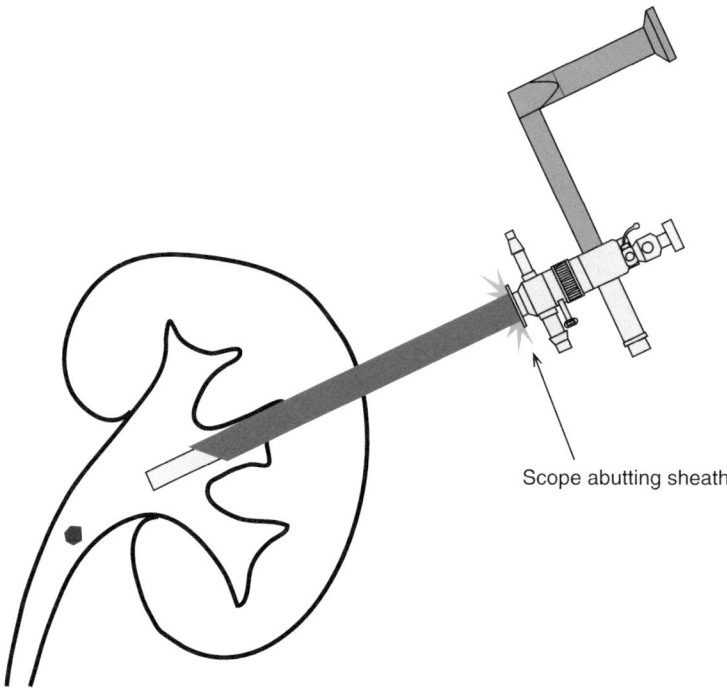

Fig. 67 Deep insertion of the nephroscope may advance the Amplatz sheath without the surgeon being aware

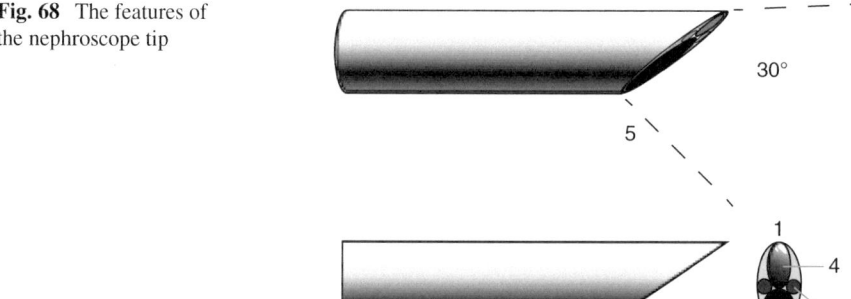

Fig. 68 The features of the nephroscope tip

This is considerably worse when a guide wire is also inside the sheath.

Note that when holding the telescope, instead of the camera, and rotating the nephroscope, it is easy to become disorientated.

Amplatz Sheath

Note that the inner diameter of the Amplatz sheath is essentially the same as the outer diameter of its dilator, so they fit together snugly.

Note that the leading end of an Amplatz sheath is oval. Therefore, it will allow a stone to enter the tip of the sheath that is larger than the diameter of the Amplatz.

Camera

Note that the camera needs to be maintained in the same position (I hold the camera left handed) so that when the scope is rotated with the right-hand instruments, there is no loss of orientation.

Whenever one is finding orientation confusing during nephroscopy, stop and remove the nephroscope and reorientate oneself outside the sheath. Then reintroduce the nephroscope.

Stone Grasping Instruments

Graspers

Alligator Forceps

These have a "scissor handle" which opens and closes the distally hinged jaws (Fig. 69).

The jaws are small and open outwards in a "V". They have a small, relatively fragile hinge and a blunt distal nose. The jaws clamp onto stone fragments in a forward action. As a result the alligator forceps cannot grasp large fragments and may push them away as the jaws close.

The jaws of the alligator forceps are ribbed; they are very effective at removing small stone fragments of 4 mm or less.

The jaws are narrow and so cannot grasp or extract clots effectively.

As the jaws are hinged and the proximal handles are strong, grasping large stones can easily break the hinge (which is expensive!).

Due to the hinge action, the alligator forceps jaws can open in small spaces, even within the ureter, as neither the shaft of the instrument nor nephroscope has to be moved for them to open.

The tips of the jaws are non-pointed and smooth, so they can be inserted atraumatically into parenchyma and opened under vision to separate the parenchyma and develop an atraumatic nephrostomy track (very useful in the scenario when a dilator cannot be fully inserted into a calyx)

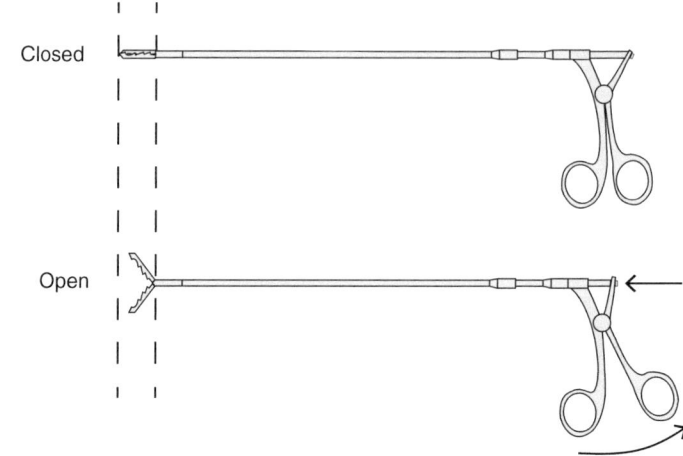

Fig. 69 The jaws of the alligator forceps.

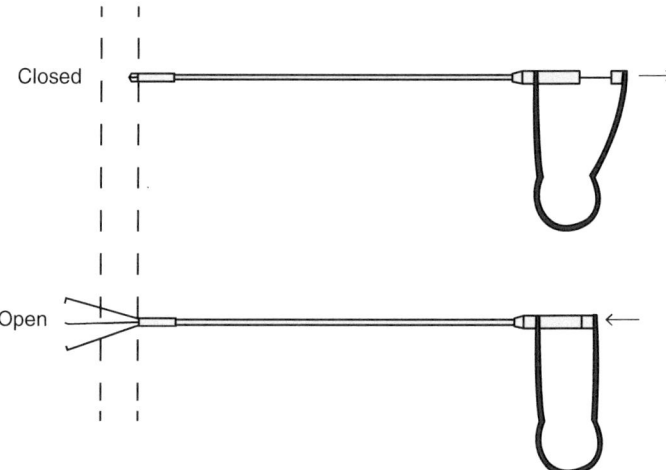

Fig. 70 The tines of the tri-radiate graspers

Triradiate Forceps

Note that these have a simple spring mechanism with no hinge joints. They are easily sterilised, cheap and strong (Fig. 70).

Stones are grasped by sharp retro-orientated tines. The tines fan out widely to entrap a stone and hold it by retracting backwards towards the operator.

Tines will grasp larger stone fragments than alligator forceps.

The tines are sharp and backward facing and can easily perforate the collecting system. They can tear and lacerate the kidney or collecting system during closure or manipulation.

Fig. 71 Comparison of the Alligator and Tri-radiate forceps when deployed

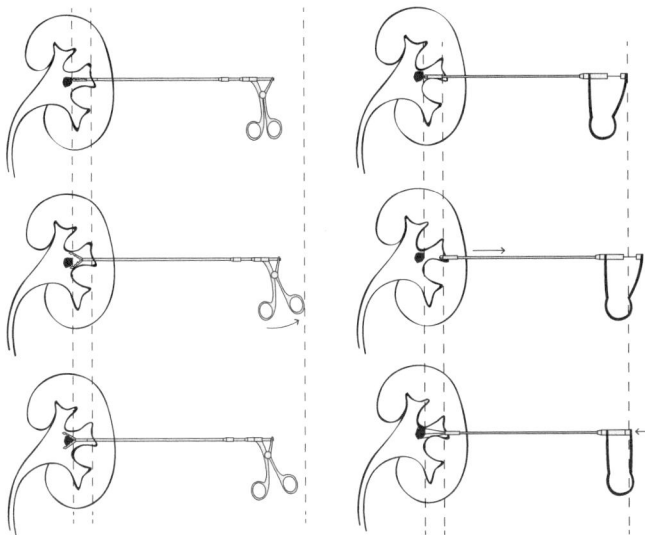

As the tines are shaped and in effect function similarly to a fish hook, should they perforate the collecting system, they can be very difficult and traumatic to disengage.

To embrace and grasp a calculus, the tines have to pass the stone for up to a centimetre. If that is not possible (such as where the stone is against the wall of the pelvis), then the shaft of the triradiate grasper needs to be retracted, and usually as a result so does the nephroscope. Therefore the application of the triradiate grasper is restricted to stones in open cavities (Fig. 71).

In practice triradiate forceps have limited use in confined spaces, such as calyces, and can be quite dangerous in the ureter, because they can easily perforate the wall.

The triradiate tines do not oppose to each other as effectively as alligator forceps, so they are inefficient for removing small fragments. Particles <4 mm slip out between the tines.

As with alligator forceps, the triradiate forceps are very inefficient at holding or extracting clot.

Ureteric Basket

Ureteric baskets are designed for use in the ureter, where the stone is immobilised. The basket needs to pass the stone and entrap the stone during retraction and closure.

It is difficult to basket a stone in an open space (such as the bladder or the renal pelvis) because the stones tend to flip out during basket closure, whereas they are immobilised in the ureter by contact with the ureteric walls.

More recent basket designs are improving the ability to basket within the kidney, especially with flexible endoscopy.

Amplatz Sheaths

The characteristics of the distal ends of the Amplatz sheath have already been described, as well the potential to cut tissues.

Note that when the proximal end of a nephroscope is in contact with the base of the Amplatz sheath, the inner opening of the sheath is proximal to the nephroscope lens and therefore invisible to the surgeon (Fig. 72).

As a result, advancement of the nephroscope in this situation will advance the Amplatz sheath. This can be dangerous when retrieving stones in the upper ureter. As the scope is advanced into the upper ureter, the sheath can lacerate or amputate the pelviureteric junction (Fig. 73).

Note that the proximal end of an Amplatz sheath is square. In obese patients, or where the sheath is inserted deeply (e.g. horseshoe kidney), the Amplatz sheath can slip under the skin. It may then be extremely difficult to retrieve.

Amplatz Modifications

(a) "Short Amplatz" (Fig. 74)

This is a useful modification for antegrade ureteroscopy with a nephroscope. By splitting the proximal end of the Amplatz sheath with scissors, to fashion 2–3-cm "pull-apart flaps", and maintaining those with artery forceps (Fig. 75), the Amplatz sheath cannot be pushed under the skin, nor can it be advanced further into the kidney or pelvis when retrieving a very distal stone (Fig. 76).

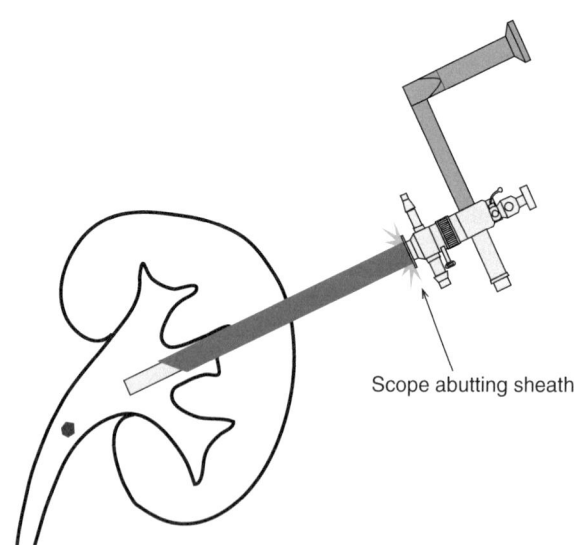

Fig. 72 Inadvertent advancement of the Amplatz sheath by the surgeon

Appendix II: PCNL Workshop

Fig. 73 Amplatz trauma resulting from inadvertent displacement of the sheath

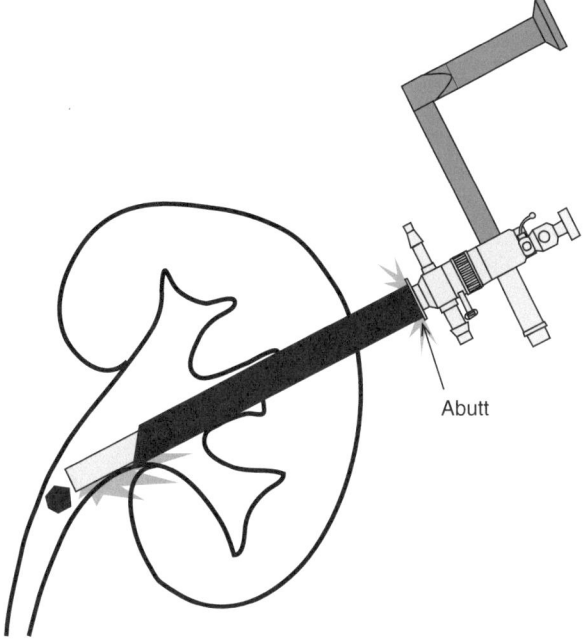

Over-advancement of the tip of the Amplatz sheath by the nephroscope unknowingly pushing the proximal end of Amplatz sheath

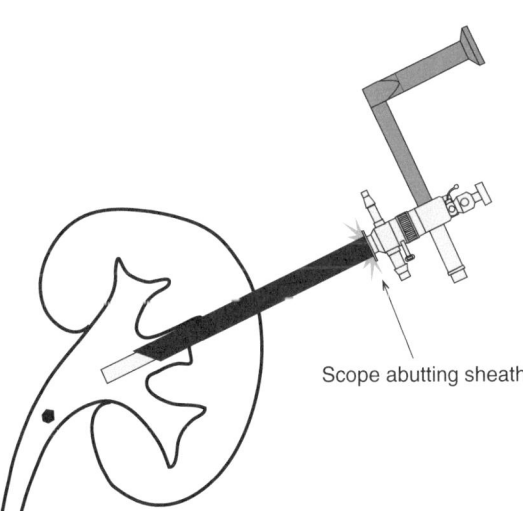

Fig. 74 If the outer end of the sheath is in contact with the endoscope, the sheath can be split

Fig. 75 Creation of a "short sheath"

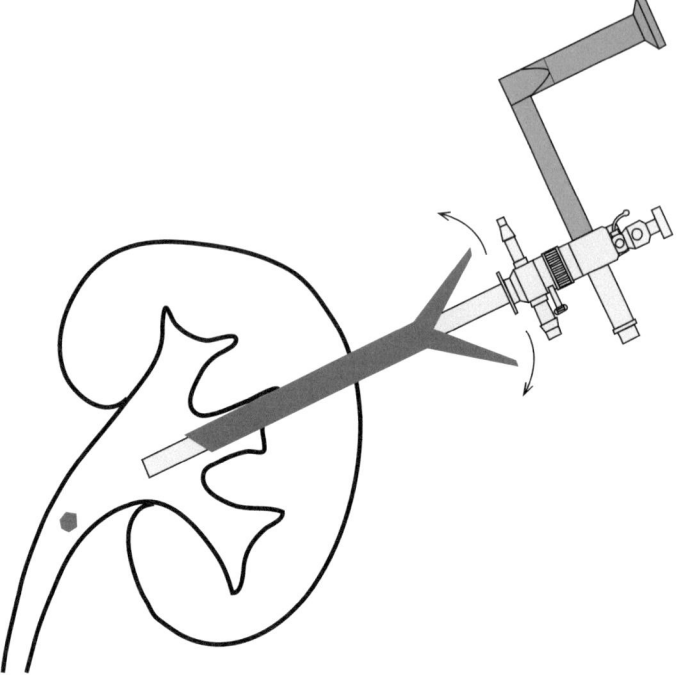

Fig. 76 Peel away the flaps to the skin edge to advance the nephroscope

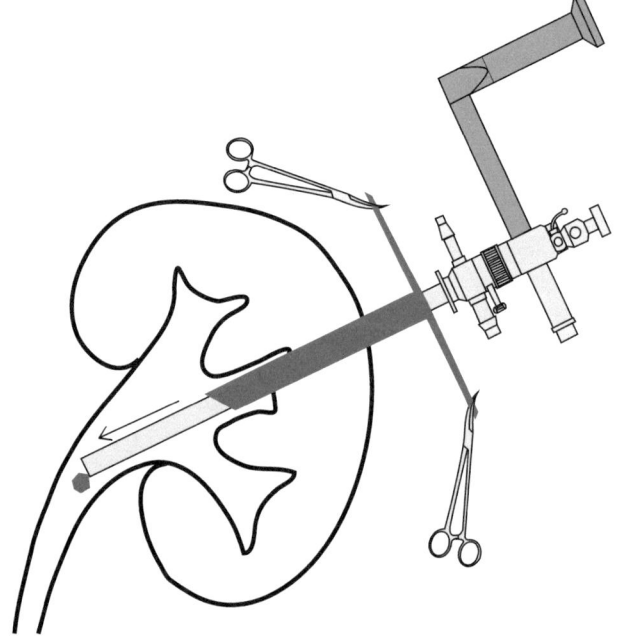

(b) "Long Amplatz"

In obese patients and in horseshoe kidneys where the nephrocutaneous track is long, a "long Amplatz" sheath can be helpful. It limits the excursion of the tip of a rigid nephroscope. In the scenario of a horseshoe kidney, the "long Amplatz" provides an excellent conduit for flexible nephroscopy and laser lithotripsy.

(c) "Peel away" sheath technique

This is a particularly useful technique to remove a sheath after a nephrostomy or stent has been placed under vision. The sheath is removed without trauma to the kidney or displacement of the nephrostomy.

Lithotrite

Ultrasound/Sonotrode

The sonotrode is a hollow metal lithotrite. It vibrates and so fragments stones using a "jack hammer" mechanism.

The sonotrode does not cause physical damage to tissues. It heats up extremely quickly, due to the energy produced by the probe vibrations. As a result the sonotrode must only be used with cooling saline irrigation and suction through the probe

The saline suction also assists by aspirating small stone particles of 2 mm or less.

If irrigation is lost, the probe can rapidly "burn out".

The vibrations from the probe can be felt by placing a probe on your finger in a beaker of water on the lowest power setting.

Note that when applying the sonotrode to chalk stone dummies under water, the sonotrode "drills" the stones, rather than shatters them (because of its low frequency and low impact vibrations).

Also note that the stone has to be immobilised for fragmentation to occur. If it is mobile, the vibrations are ineffective.

Pneumatic Lithotrite

This is a simple metal rod attached to a proximal pneumatic cylinder. No suction is required. The rod does not heat up with use. The rod is can be resterilised and does not wear out.

As long as the probe is not applied forcibly to the stone, the pneumatic pulses do not injure soft tissues. This can be tested with your finger under water and single-low-dose pressure pulses generated.

The pneumatic probe fragments calculi into large pieces.

The pneumatic probe will fragment much harder and dense stones than the ultrasound probe.

For effective fragmentation using the pneumatic lithotripter, the stone also needs to be immobilised. Pressure on the stone may result in displacement along the ureter or around the kidney when the pulses are applied.

Lithotrites

Set up the ultrasound sonotrode with the suction pump and water irrigation.

Switch on the ultrasound probe for 2–3 s and feel the heat generated. Attach the suction and saline, activate the sonotrode and note that it now remains cool.

Place the ultrasound probe on low power on the finger under water, to feel the vibrations, and confirm it is atraumatic.

Apply the probe through a nephroscope to chalk to reduce it to small fragments.

Using the triradiate and alligator forceps, remove large and small chalk fragments through a nephroscope. Observe the ease which the alligator forceps grasp small stones and the strength of the triradiate grasper for larger stones.

Note that if you place a large chalk dummy in the jaws of the alligator forceps near the hinge, closing the forceps will advance the stone out of its grip.

Note that small stones (3–4 mm) are easily picked up by the alligator forceps between using the distal two thirds of the jaws.

Observe that neither the nephroscope nor the alligator forceps need to be advanced or retracted to fully open and deploy the alligator jaws.

Use the forceps as above through a nephroscope to pick up small and large "calculi" fragmented within the beakers.

Triradiate Forceps

Observe that the jaws need to advance away from the nephroscope and instrument shaft beyond the stone to open the tines. Observe that the tines are very sharp and point backward towards the surgeon, so they function similarly to "fish hooks". The tines need pass the stone to entrap it. They grip by reverse action. If they have perforated the collecting system, the reverse action can cut and lacerate the soft stones.

Pass the triradiate forceps through an Amplatz sheath and grasp a large stone dummy. Note that it can be pulled into the oval opening but then not extracted along the shaft of the Amplatz sheath, due to the disparity in cross section between the circular shaft and the oval opening.

Summary

Alligator forceps are easy and fast for the extraction of small stone fragments and very effective within the small confined spaces of the kidney, the calyces or the ureter.

However, they are fragile, are expensive and have difficulty holding larger stones, and if used with force, the hinge joint will break.

Fig. 77 Creation of a "short sheath" for deep nephroscopy and ureteroscopy

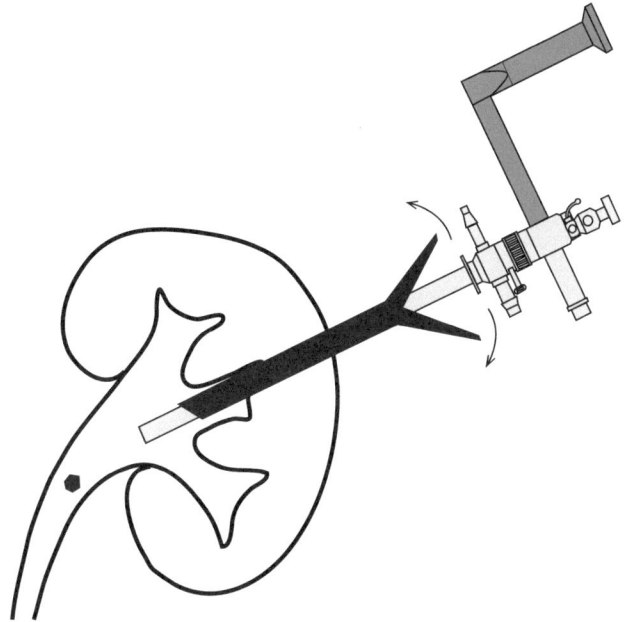

Triradiate forceps are simple, cheap, strong and good for removing large stone fragments. However, small fragments can fall through the tines, and perforation can result in ureteric or pelvic trauma. A large space is required for deployment so the safe use of the triradiate forceps is restricted in small and angled spaces.

Versions of the Amplatz Sheath

Short Amplatz Sheath (Fig. 77)

Take an Amplatz sheath, divide it with heavy scissors at the proximal end for 2–3 cm, and create a "short sheath" by attaching artery forceps to either side of the division.

Then convert the short sheath to a peel away sheath by pulling the artery forceps apart completely to split the sheath into two halves (Fig. 78).

Creation of a Long Sheath

Take a 24-French dilator, place its appropriate sheath over it, and then take a sheath from a 28-French dilator, jam the oval end over the proximal end of the 24 sheath, keeping the 24 sheath flush with the dilator (Fig. 79). Then take a nephroscope and place it so that the tip of the nephroscope has at least a 1.5-cm distal excursion from the operating end of the Amplatz sheath (Fig. 80).

Mark the proximal end where the hilt of the nephroscope abuts the French sheath,

Fig. 78 The "peel away" technique for removal of the Amplatz sheath after inserting a nephrostomy

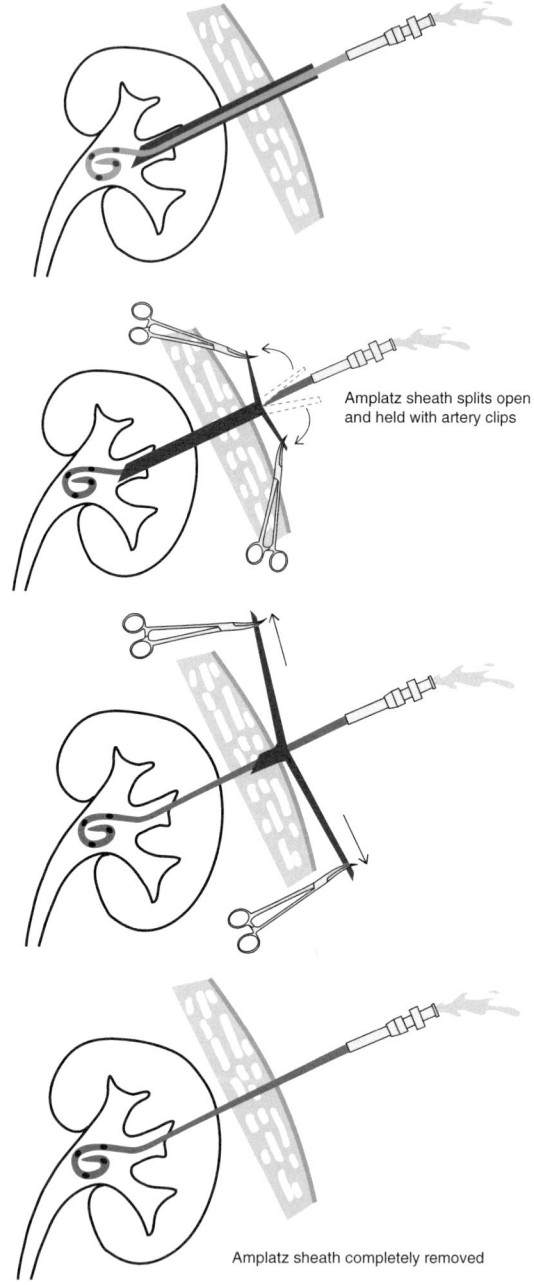

Appendix II: PCNL Workshop 247

Divide the sheath at this mark with a scalpel. The two sheaths will stay together and act as one. This long sheath can be very effective for PCNL in horseshoe kidneys (Fig. 81).

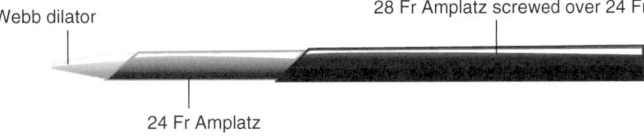

Fig. 79 Creation of a "long sheath" - screw a larger Amplatz sheath over the initial sheath to obtain a tight fit

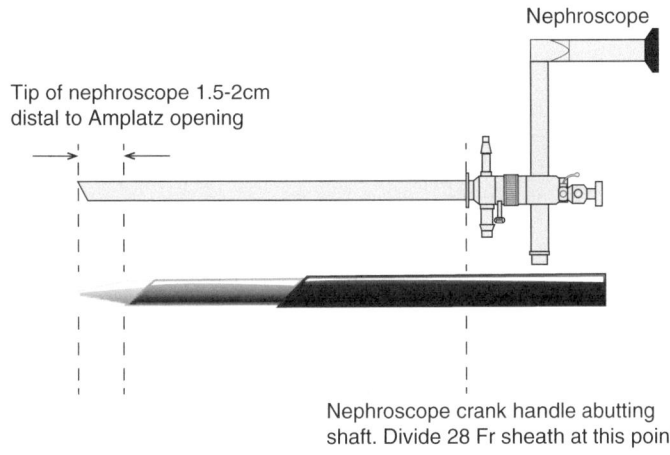

Fig. 80 The sheath is measured against the nephrostomy to ensure there is at least 1.2-2 cm distal extension of the nephroscope internally

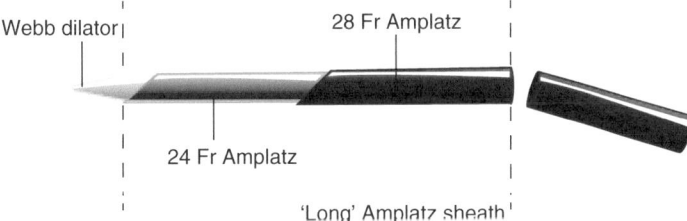

Fig. 81 Perpendicular division of the sheath with a heavy scalpel blade

Glossary and Definitions

A

Air Contrast Technique The injection of air through a retrograde catheter to identify a posterior calyx in a hydronephrosis prior to renal puncture when contrast alone is unable to identify the calyx.

Alligator Forceps Hinged grasping forceps for use through a nephroscope.

Amplatz Sheath A circular synthetic tube placed over a dilator into the kidney to form a conduit from the skin to the kidney for surgery.

Arteriovenous Fistula An abnormal arteriovenous connection within the kidney following PCNL.

B

Basket A metal or newer material such as nitinol spiral or rounded wire trap that can be passed through a fine catheter and opened under vision or radiological control to retrieve calculi.

Balloon The retaining device on a urethral catheter or a sausage-like expansion balloon on a percutaneous track dilator.

Beanbag A vinyl bag with plastic beads attached to suction, upon which the patient is placed for PCNL. The air is evacuated which maintains the shape to support the patient. Particularly useful for patients with musculoskeletal deformities.

C

Calyceal Diverticulum A congenital pouch extending from a calyx, usually rounded with a stork-like neck. Urine refluxes into a calyceal diverticulum from the calyx but is not secreted by the renal parenchyma into the diverticulum.

CT/KUB Computed tomography of the kidney, ureter and bladder without contrast.

CT/IVP Computed tomography using contrast media of the kidney, ureter and bladder performed in phases.
 (a) Arterial
 (b) Excretory to outline the kidney and the collecting system

Cope A self-retaining fine nephrostomy tube maintained within the kidney by a loop formed by pulling on a very fine string through the nephrostomy catheter.

D

Dilator (Renal) Various dilators are used to dilate a track from the skin to the collecting system of the kidney through the body wall and renal parenchyma. These include:
 (a) Serial Amplatz dilators
 (b) Alken telescoping metal car aerial dilators
 (c) Balloon dilators
 (d) Single-stage dilators, e.g. Webb and mini-perc

E

Endopyelotomy The endoscopic incision of a pelvic ureteric junction stricture, through a nephrostomy or ureteroscopically.

ESWL Extracorporeal shock wave lithotripsy, contact-free fragmentation of urinary calculi by externally applied shock waves.

Endoscopic Nephrotomy The creation of a nephrotomy under vision using alligator forceps through a nephroscope passed through an Amplatz sheath from the outer border of the renal capsule to the calyx.

F

"Flash Sign" The sudden appearance of methylene blue and contrast into a syringe upon withdrawing the nephrostomy needle sheath while applying gentle aspiration after a puncture has transgressed a calyx.

French Guage (Charriere) The circumference or length of the external border of surgical items such as a urethral catheter, a nephrostomy tube or renal dilator.
FUL Flexible ureteroscopic laser lithotripsy of a calculus.
Foley A self-retaining urethral balloon catheter which can also be used as a nephrostomy.

G

Golf T Introducer A device for straightening and introducing floppy and J-tipped guide wires into a catheter or nephrostomy needle sheath.
Guide Wires Guide wires can be metallic, solid or coated with hydrophilic material. They may be straight and have a floppy or a "J tip". Guide wires are radio-opaque and pass through ureteric catheters. Various other catheters with dilators can be passed over guide wires.

H

Hydrophilic Guide Wire (Slippery) A guide wire covered in hydrophilic materials so that they become exceedingly slippery once wet.

I

ICU Intensive care unit.
II Image intensifier.

K

Knife Usually applied to an endoscopic knife. A "hot knife" carries an electric current and can cut and coagulate. A "cold knife" has no current. It cuts directly via a sharp edge.
Sickle Knife This is a cold knife which instead of cutting straight ahead is "fish-hooked" in shape and cuts by withdrawal towards the surgeon.

L

Laser The commonest used laser for stone fragmentation as the Holmium-Yag laser, especially for flexible ureteroscopic laser lithotripsy or flexible nephroscopy.

Lens The optical lens of a ureteroscope, nephroscope or cystoscope which may be angled at the end. An oblique lens gives a wider view, requiring rotation of the instrument. A zero lens gives a straight head view, most useful when looking along a tubular structure.

M

Malecot A self-retaining catheter without a balloon is fashioned so that when inserted over an internal stylet, the head of the catheter will form lateral wings so that it is self-retaining once the stylet is removed.

Methylene Blue Sign The nephroscope appearance of saline and methylene blue injected through a retrograde catheter, which enables the surgeon to identify the direction of the calyx leading to the renal pelvis.

Mini-PCNL The description given to smaller nephroscopic instruments and their application through nephrostomies of less than 20 French, modelled originally on paediatric nephroscopes.

Modified Calyceal Universal Guide Wire A wire placed, usually after multiple punctures into the kidney, through one calyx which is then grasped within the renal pelvis and retracted through a separate calyx to provide a wire for dilation.

Monitor In endourology this refers to the image intensifier screen viewed by the surgeon.

N

Nephroscope A telescope used for looking into the kidney at either open or percutaneous renal surgery. May be rigid or flexible.

Nephrostomy A tube draining urine from the collecting system of the kidney to the skin, usually self-retaining.

Nephrostomy "(Tubeless)" A double J stent inserted into the kidney following a percutaneous operation without an external nephrostomy.

Needle Tip These may be diamond shaped, in which case they tend to track straight ahead, or bevelled and angled, in which case as they pass through the body tissues, they will tend to curve with respect to the angle of the tip of the needle.

O

Offset The rigid nephroscope has an offset lens; in other words, the lens comes in either at a right angle or an angle to the rigid nephroscope, allowing for a straight instrument and irrigation channel for rigid instruments.

P

PCN Percutaneous nephrostomy.
PCNL Percutaneous nephrolithotomy.
PCRS Percutaneous renal surgery.
Puncture "(Y)" and "Target" Direct punctures into individual calyces. The "Y" puncture from an adjacent nephrostomy track, the "target" puncture from a new nephrostomy track.
Pyelolysis The original name given by Dr John Wickham to endoscopic pyeloplasty performed percutaneously.

R

Radical Nephrectomy Complete ablation of the kidney and surrounding tissues for cancer.
Retroperitoneal Guide Wire Technique The technique of passing a guide wire alongside a stone and through the kidney into the retroperitoneal tissues to stabilise it and so allow a dilatation directly onto the calculus.
RGC Retrograde catheter.
RGP Retrograde pyelogram.

S

Single Stage Originally this was a term used to describe percutaneous nephrolithotomy, in which the nephrostomy and the PCNL were performed synchronously under the same anaesthetic.
Single-Stage Dilator A dilator which will create a nephrocutaneous track by a single passage (Webb SSD, mini-perc dilators).
Sickle Knife A cold knife used with a visual urethrotome to cut a stricture in a pelviureteric junction obstruction (endoscopic pyeloplasty).
Stent An internal ureteric splint from the kidney to the bladder, with a self-retaining memory loop at either end to maintain the position of the stent.
Stone dusting The process of stone breakdown with a laser fibre or lithoclast set to reduce the stone edge to very fine particles which flush out of a nephrostomy or down the ureter without the need for basket or grasper extraction.

T

Target Another name for a single-stage dilator, or the direct passage of a needle and dilators into a single calyx.

Tine The grasping prongs of the triradiate forceps which angle back towards the surgeon.

Track Used in percutaneous renal surgery to describe the nephrocutaneous conduit formed by dilatation from the skin to the inner aspect of the kidney.

Tract Technically a stretch of land and urologically describes the entire urinary tract, in other words kidneys, ureter, bladder, prostate and urethra.

Triradiate Grasper A nephroscopic stone extracting instrument which is hingeless and strong with tines that radiate from the tip of the grasper to embrace the calculus and then hold it by reverse traction.

TUR Prostate Transurethral resection of the prostate.

TUR Syndrome The absorption of fluid associated with blood loss and infection and electrolyte imbalance seen with TUR prostate which can also occur with prolonged percutaneous nephrolithotomy.

Tubeless Used to describe post-operative scenario following a PCNL where there is no nephrostomy, just an internal double J stent.

U

UGW Universal guide wire. A guide wire entering the urethra through the bladder and ureter and exiting through the kidney and the skin.

URS Ureteroscopy.

Ureteroscope A flexible or rigid instrument passed from the bladder up to the ureter or through a nephrostomy down the ureter (antegrade ureteroscopy).

V

Visual Urethrotome An endoscopic working element with a cold knife for cutting urethral strictures which can be used with the sickle knife for percutaneous endopyelotomy.

Vacuum Cleaner Effect During "Mini-PCNL" due to the sheath geometry and withdrawal of the nephroscope during continuous irrigation, a vortex develops in the lumen of the working sheath. This acts as a vacuum so that stone dust and fragments are flushed out of the sheath without the need for stone graspers or baskets.

Y

"Y" (Puncture) The puncture of an adjacent calyx following an initial puncture into a closely adjourning calyx, using the existing body wall track.

Index

A
Amplatz trauma
 lost, 178
 sites of, 177
Anaesthetist, 19
Anderson-Hynes pyeloplasty, 10

B
Bleeding, 183–184
Blood supply, PCNL complications, 170
Bowel
 dilator trauma
  during track dilation, 173–174
 needle puncture of, 173
 perforation, 172, 174

C
Calculi within calyceal diverticulae
 anticipated difficulties, 137–138
 drainage, 144–145
 guide wire, 144
 puncture, 138
 stone removal, 144
 surgery
  CT-IVU, 138–139
  needle puncture, 139
  options, 140
 "Y" puncture technique, 141–142
  application of, 142–143
Calyceal diverticulae (CD), 7, 53, 112, 137–139
Calyceal lumen, 8

Calyceal spasm, 8
Calyces, 4
Calyx
 needle puncture, 5
 previous renal surgery, 146
 renal scarring, 147
Capsular needle puncture, 3
Collecting system, PCNL
  complications, 170
Complex anatomy, 112–114
Complex calculi, 111
Complex recurrent infection calculi, urine infection
 difficulties and problems, 135
 stone removal, indication
  aims of treatment, 135
  parenteral antibiotics, 136
  pre-admission, 135–136
  preoperative preparation, 136
"Cope" loop nephrostomy, 105
 UGW, 107–108
"Cope" nephrostomy
 insertion following PCNL, 106–107
 suture, 109
 tube to skin, 108–109

D
Deep vein thrombosis (DVT), 52, 185

E
Electrohydraulic probes, 97
Endoscopic pyeloplasty, 53

Equipment requirements
  access, 22
  antibiotics, 26
  artery forceps, 23
  blankets and drapes, 26
  C-ARM, 21–22
  hydrophilic or "slippery" guide wires, 22–23
  imaging, 21
  operation table, 20
  patient drape, 26
  patient positioning, 20–22
  prophylaxis, 26
  retrograde catheter, 23
  scalpel, 27
  urethral catheter, 23–26
Extracorporal shockwave lithotripsy (ESWL), 50, 91, 103, 111, 112, 116, 151, 182, 185

F
Flexible ureterorenoscopic laser lithotripsy (FURS), 48, 49, 52, 103, 111, 116, 117, 151, 152
Foley catheter, 105
Forceps trauma, 178–179

G
Gerota's fascia, 6, 12, 13, 16
Guide wires
  Amplatz serial exchange dilators, 28
  Amplatz sheath, 32–35
  balloon dilators, 29–30
  Golf Tee introducer, 27
  intracorporal stone fragmentation, 37
  irrigation fluid, 36
  "mini perc" dilators, 31–32
  nephroscopes, 36–37
  nephrostomy track dilators, 28
  percutaneous endoscopic pyloplasty, 39–40
  pneumatic ballistic lithotrites (lithoclast), 37–38
  puncture needle, 35–36
  sonotrode, 38–39
  telescopic "car aerial" dilators (alken), 28–29
  types, 27
  webb single-stage dilator, 30–31

H
Horseshoe kidney
  collecting system, 17
  paraspinal muscles, 17
  pelvis and pelviureteric junction, 17
  preoperative planning
    CT-IVU, 150–151
    endoscopy, 151
    operative plan, 151
    puncture, 151
    track, 151
  vasculature, 16–17

I
Infection-related staghorn calculus
  aim, 115
  CT-IVP, 116–117
  endoscopic nephrotomy, 125–128
  potential problems, 116
  preoperative tests, 116
  punctures for, 118–124
  pyonephrosis, 117
  removal, 129–134
  treatment and precautions, 116
Infundibula, 4
Infundibular tears, 180–182
Infundibulum, 1, 2
Intrarenal anatomy, PCNL complications, 170

K
Kidney. *See also* Horseshoe kidney
  horseshoe kidney, 16–17
  PCNL complications, 169

L
Langer's line, 15
Large hydronephrosis, percutaneous puncture of
  operative technique, 161
  plan, 161
Larger dilators separate, 9
Large staghorn calculus, 53
Large upper ureteric calculus
  antegrade PCNL to remove, 152
  preoperative planning
    amplatz trauma, 159–160
    CT-IVP, 152–153
    procedure, 153–157
    three-wire antegrade ureteroscopy technique, 157–158
Laser, 97
Lithotrite
  pneumatic lithoclast, 99–100
  ultrasonic lithotrite (sonotrode), 99
"Lost" calculi, 181–182
Lost nephrostomy, 108
Lost nephrostomy track, 182

Index

M
Medical assistant, 20
Medical personnel
  anaesthetist, 19
  assistant, 20
  nursing, 19–20
  radiographer, 20
  surgeon, 20
  theatre technician/orderly, 20
Microvasculature, 1, 2

N
Needle puncture
  bowel, 173
  calculi within calyceal
    diverticulae, 139
  calyx, 5
  capsular, 3
  guide wires, 35–36
Nephrectomy, 47, 48, 52
Nephrolithotomy, 47, 52, 93
Nephroscope and sheath movements, 9
Nephroscopy and stone removal
  blood clots, 92–93
  clot removal, 93
  lithotrite, 99–100
  nephroscopes, 91–92
  plan, 90–91
  sonotrode, 98–99
  stone fragmentation, 97–98
  universal guide wire (UGW), 93–97
Nephrostogram, 110
Nephrostomy
  "cope" loop, 104–105
  post-operative care of, 109
  post PCNL, 104
  puncture
    guide wire kinking during
      dilation, 172
    neighbouring organs, damage,
      172–174
    renal vein or IVC puncture, 175
  types, 104
Nursing, 19–20

O
Obese patient, horseshoe kidney, 53
Obese patients, 147–148
  preoperative planning
    CT/IVU, 148
    nephroscope, 148
    sheath, 148–149

P
PCN. See Percutaneous nephrostomy
  (PCN)
PCNL. See Percutaneous nephrolithotomy
  (PCNL)
Pelviureteric junction, 1, 2, 10, 151
Percutaneous access, anatomy
  bad track, 11–12
  body wall, 12–15
  good track, 10–11
  horseshoe kidney, 16–17
  lumbodorsal fascia, 15
  renal, 1–10
Percutaneous endopyelotomy (pyeloplasty)
  indications, 161–162
  operative plan
    air contrast technique, 164–165
    CT-IVP, 163
    equipment, 163
    percutaneous puncture, 163–164
    previous surgery, 162
  operative technique, 166–167
  supracostal punctures, 167
  precautions
    bleeding from intercostal
      vessel, 167
    pneumothorax, 168
  technique and difficulties, 162
Percutaneous nephrolithotomy (PCNL)
  advanced skills requirement, 115
  body wall anatomical
    relationships for, 13
  complications of
    anatomical factors, 169–171
    forceps trauma, 178–179
    infundibular tears, 180–182
    nephrostomy puncture, 172–175
    renal pelvis perforation, 179–180
    track dilation, 175–178
    urinary tract infection and septicaemia,
      182–185
  consent, 52
  contraindications to, 49
  and ESWL, 50
  indications for, 47–49
  preoperative investigations, 51–52
  preoperative theatre preparation, 52–53
  punctures for, 12
  stone clearance, 104
  stone extraction for
    alligator forceps, 100–101
    baskets, 102–103
    instruments, 100
    triradiate forceps, 101–102

Percutaneous nephrolithotomy (PCNL) (cont.)
   track, 3
   track dilatation, 83
      aim, 84
      kinked guide wire, 86
      lumbodorsal fascia, 87
      nephrostomy track, body wall component of, 87
      principles, 84–86
      skin, 87
   track dilation
      dilator, 88–89
      guide wire, 88
   track size, 84
Percutaneous nephrostomy (PCN)
   lithotomy position, 64–65
   prone position of patient, 66–68
   puncture technique, 56–64
   radiological nephrostomy (RN), 56, 81–82
   skinny needle surgical nephrostomy (SNSN), 55
   surgical nephrostomy (SN), 55
   theatre set-up
      calyceal puncture, 79–81
      needle placement, 74–79
      needle, puncture and insertion of, 73
      patient and equipment set-up, 68–69
      patient draping, 69–70
      percutaneous renal puncture, 70–72
      personnel and equipment, positioning of, 68
Percutaneous puncture, 163–164
Pneumatic ballistic lithotrites (lithoclast)
   advantages, 38
   disadvantages, 38
   indications, 37–38
Pneumothorax, 183
PUJ avulsion, 180
Punctures. *See also* Needle puncture
   calculi within calyceal diverticulae, 138
   horseshoe kidney, 151
   infection-related staghorn calculus, 118–124
   nephrostomy
      guide wire kinking during dilation, 172
      neighbouring organs, damage, 172–174
      PCNL complications of, 172–175
      renal vein or IVC puncture, 175
   PCN
      calyceal puncture, 79–81
      needle, puncture and insertion of, 73
      percutaneous renal puncture, 70–72
      puncture technique, 56–64
   PCNL, 12

R
Radiographer, 20
Radiological nephrostomy (RN), 56, 81–82
Renal arterial vasculature, 10
Renal calculi, treatment of, 48
Renal capsule, 7
Renal parenchyma, 1
Renal pelvis, 1, 2
Renal pelvis contract, 4
Renal pelvis perforation, 179–180
Renal puncture, 7. *See also* Needle puncture; Punctures
Renal stone disease, 47
Residual calculi, 184–185
Retrograde ureteric catheter (RGC), 22
Routine PCNL. *See* Percutaneous nephrolithotomy (PCNL)

S
Segmental renal blood supply, 10
"Slippery" wires, 23
Sonotrode, 99
Sonotrode trauma, 180–181
Spastic contraction, 4
Stone clearance, 103–104
Stone extraction
   alligator forceps, 100–101
   baskets, 102–103
   instruments, 100
   triradiate forceps, 101–102
Stone fragmentation
   aims of, 97–98
   alternative energy sources for, 97
   optimal lithotrites, 97
Stone grasping instruments
   chest drains, 46
   cope nephrostomy, 44
   Foley balloon catheters, 44
   graspers
      alligator forceps, 40
      triradiate forceps, 40–42
   nephrostomies, 42–43
   penrose drain, 45
   tubeless nephrostomy, 46
   yeates drain, 45
Stone removal
   blood clots, 92–93
   calculi within calyceal diverticulae, 144
   clot removal, 93
   complex recurrent infection calculi, urine infection
      aims of treatment, 135
   lithotrite, 99–100

nephroscopes, 91–92
plan, 90–91
sonotrode, 98–99
stone fragmentation, 97–98
universal guide wire (UGW), 93–97
Supracostal punctures, 167
Surgeon, 20

T
Theatre, additional equipment
  aims of surgery, 136
  ileal conduit, 137
  surgical approach, 137
Theatre technician/orderly, 20
Track and kidney dilation, 89–90
Track dilatation, 83
  aim, 84
  kinked guide wire, 86
  lumbodorsal fascia, 87
  nephrostomy track, body wall component of, 87
  principles, 84–86
  skin, 87
Track dilation
  complications
    calyx, 176
    lost track during dilation, 175–176
  dilator, 88–89
  guide wire, 88

Triradiate forceps, 178–179
Tubeless nephrostomy, 106
Tube nephrostomy (splinted), 105

U
Universal guide wire (UGW), 22
  advantages of, 96–97
  "cope" loop nephrostomy, 107–108
  creation of, 94–95
  skin to urethral meatus, 93
Upper ureteric calculus, 53, 151
Ureter, 1, 2
Urethral catheter, 16 Fr Foley
  contrast, 25–26
  functions, 23–25
Urinary tract infection and septicaemia
  intraoperative sepsis, 182
  post-operative fever, 183
  pre-operatively, 182

V
Vasculature, 16–17

Y
"Y" puncture technique, 141–143

If you have any concerns about our products,
you can contact us on
ProductSafety@springernature.com

In case Publisher is established outside the EU,
the EU authorized representative is:
**Springer Nature Customer Service Center GmbH
Europaplatz 3, 69115 Heidelberg, Germany**

Printed by Libri Plureos GmbH
in Hamburg, Germany